"I have had the good fortune to practice yoga, Tai Chi and Qi Gong with Karen and Shirley during the past twenty years. They so expertly guide their students to develop proficiency and awareness of the movements involved in the practices. At the same time, they promote an understanding of the relationship of these movements to the body's optimum health."

Penny Kelly, Mill Valley, Ca

All About Balance

Maintain and Improve balance for Active, Healthy Aging

A BLEND OF EAST AND WEST
PRINCIPLES AND PRACTICES

Karen Dockstader and Shirley Dockstader

All About Balance

Copyright © 2025 by Karen Dockstader and Shirley Dockstader

ISBN 979-8-9991383-0-9 (print)
ISBN 979-8-9991383-1-6 (ebook)

Cover design: Karen Dockstader
Photographer: Covey Cowan, Sam Cowan, Lea Itkin
Interior layout: Val Sherer, Personalized Publishing Services
Copy editing: Ashley Brown

All rights reserved.
Printed in the United States of America

We dedicate this book to our beloved students who made this all possible, and the masterful teachers from whom we have had the privilege to learn.

We also thank Don Goewey, author, and Jamie Wallach M.D., who offered encouragement and feedback when most needed.

For more information and videos visit:
seniorsinbalance.com

"Balance is the underlying foundation of longevity in all that exists"

Anodea Judith

Contents

Foreword ix

Introduction 1

I. What Do We Mean By Balance? 7

II. The Body Systems 'Changes as We Age' and
'What we can do' 13

    Musculoskeletal System 18

    Neurological System 23

    Sensory Systems 32

    Subtle Energy System 42

III. The Contributions to Balance of Eastern Practices 49

IV. The contributions to Balance of Western Mind/Body Methods 59

V. The Essence of Practice 63

VI. The Structure of a Class or Personal Practice. 69

VII. The Basic Movements 77

VIII. And Finally 151

    References 155

    About the Authors 160

Foreword

Balance is one of the most essential — and most overlooked — foundations of health. It underlies every step we take, every movement we make, and every sense of confidence we have in our bodies. Yet, despite its importance, balance is rarely studied in depth in Western medical education, leaving both physicians and patients without a systematic understanding of how it can be nurtured, maintained, and restored throughout life.

That is precisely why *All About Balance* is such an important and timely book. Drawing on decades of teaching and practice, the authors bring together the wisdom of Eastern traditions — where movement, posture, and awareness have been studied for centuries — with the rigor of Western approaches to anatomy, physiology, and rehabilitation. This unique blend of perspectives creates a guide that is both practical and profound.

For seniors in particular, the value of this work cannot be overstated. Falls are one of the greatest threats to independence and quality of life as we age, and yet the skills of balance, coordination, and mindful movement can be strengthened at any stage of life. With clear explanations and beautifully illustrated exercises, this book offers readers tools to improve stability, confidence, and overall well-being.

But *All About Balance* is not only for older adults. Physicians, physical therapists, and health professionals will also find in these pages insights that are not taught in medical school — insights that can transform their ability to help patients maintain mobility, prevent injury, and reclaim vitality.

This is more than a book of exercises; it is two lifetimes of experience distilled into a clear, accessible, and inspiring guide. By integrating Eastern and Western wisdom, the Dockstaders provide us all with a much-needed path toward steadiness — in our bodies and in our lives.

Martin L. Rossman, M.D.

Author, The Worry Solution

Mill Valley, California 2025

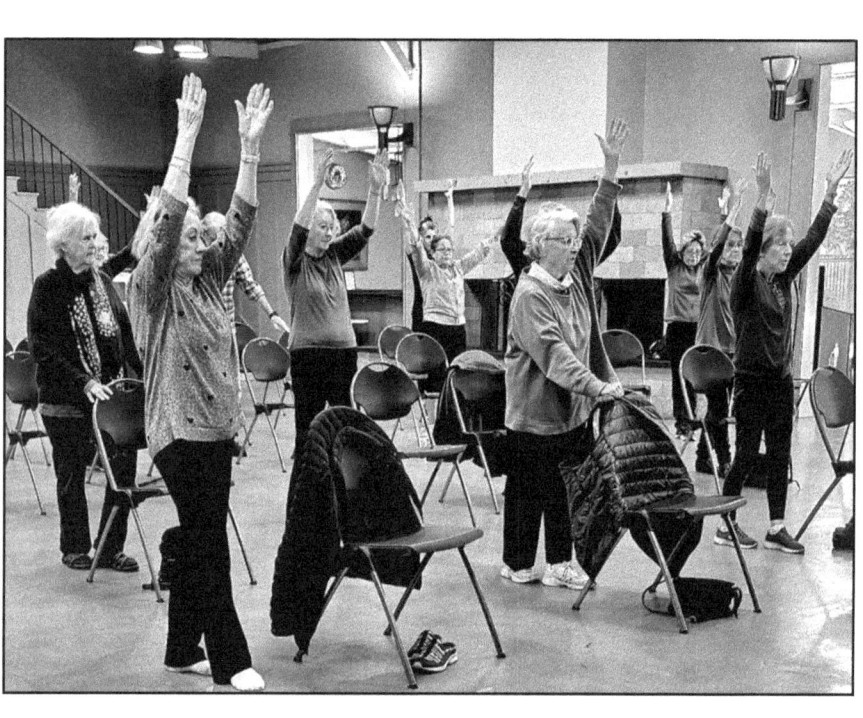

Introduction

> *"When no resistance is encountered, Qi flow is ample and harmonious and nothing restrains its natural tendency to circulate. All of the body functions are nourished without effort. The promise of circulation is that the potential of the human being may be enhanced, not by forcing it, but by simply allowing it. Remove resistance and energy flows."*
>
> Roger Janke, The Healing Promise of Qi

Aging most often creeps up on us. Like many seniors we know, you may feel as alive in spirit as you did years ago. Yet, the body has a way of reminding us of the changes we have undergone. How do we still stay vital and engaged in spite of these changes, and maintain the confidence to adapt and rebalance as time goes on? In this book we hope to address this question.

Many people are transforming their inherited ideas of what aging means and adopting instead the inspiring idea that our elder years are what we make of them. Aging with grace and resounding joy depends upon being in touch with the source that fuels and enlivens us and keeps our bodies and spirits in balance.

Working with seniors through the healing movement arts, we witness a common longing to deepen our connection with our essential selves and share that connection with others.

Once we begin to make internal connections (body, movement, breath, mind, emotions, and spirit) and acknowledge them with awareness, our practices expand beyond the forms and begin to grace our lives in every way. We can re-enter a time of innocence, curiosity, spontaneity, and openness to life. In the seniors we teacher, we have witnessed veritable wisdom as they enjoy a time in life that brings less distraction with external demands — as well as openness, gratitude, and receptivity to being present.

Balance is critical to healthy aging!

This book gives a foundation in the components of balance. It also offers a perspective of common age-related changes to balance and what we can do about it. It covers the science of balance, the ancient wisdom and the experience. This book is meant to be a resource and used in whatever way best serves you. When we are supple in life, neither resistant to nor victims of change, we have the capacity to renew and rebalance.

How does this program differ from the many existing fitness opportunities for seniors? The most important difference is in its integration of Eastern focus on internal awareness, breath, and flowing movement, with a western core strength, function, and flexibility approach to balance. Both are important.

This program complements other valuable senior fitness activities such as weight training, aerobics (walking, running, fitness machines), other sports, and deeper studies in yoga, Tai Chi, or Qigong for those who are interested.

Our aim is to address a niche that brings together pearls from each of these traditions and modalities to specifically work with balance for seniors in a gentle and accessible balance-directed format — working with all systems of the body and mind that are affected by age. Balance is mercurial. Every day is different. However, with practice and attention, we can gain greater stability and confidence, and develop a greater ability to understand and navigate change in our bodies as well as in our environment.

Our students are seniors varying in mobility and age, some well into their 90s, who are motivated to take responsibility for their health and are desirous of restoring or maintaining good balance and coordination. The truth is that balance changes begin in our 30s, and many of these principles and practices can be beneficially incorporated into one's movement practices at any age. 'The exercises can be done seated, standing, standing and holding the back of a chair, or a combination of all three.

This book should in no way replace valuable medical advice or treatment. It is meant to enhance the options and approaches to health available for seniors. Anyone uncertain about the suitability of the program for themselves should consult with their doctor.

The risk of falls for seniors is very real. One in four adults over 65 and over half of adults 80 and above fall every year. Falls are the leading cause of injury among older adults. There are of course many causes, ranging from specific medical conditions to unsupportive environmental conditions (see pages 10 & 11). Some of those causes, however, are based on common changes many of us experience as we age, which can be improved through training.

Students from our classes have told us they feel less afraid of falling, and more confident in their ability to maintain their balance. They have also expressed improvement in their mobility and level of energy. At the end of each class, the seniors leave uplifted and more relaxed. We have written this book to give a background into what we teach and why for students who may be interested in expanding their understanding, and for those who themselves may offer classes for seniors.

Karen: Building strength from the inside out

I (Karen), have experienced a number of injuries that have at times left me considering the possibility of spending the rest of my life in pain. I no longer experience that pain, and my body feels strong. The practices offered in this book have been instrumental in my own body's healing. Likewise, one of my students mentioned to me that she had an injury and surgery that never fully healed. She tried PT and other modalities but nothing seemed to help. She wanted to know why the senior class, while being so gentle, was the one thing that made a difference. Often the most seemingly subtle practices can be the most powerful. The gentle, yet nourishing practices encourage energy flow, integrity, harmony, fluidity and ultimately kindness of one's whole body, building strength from the inside out.

Shirley: Tools

I share with all of you the apprehensions of aging: Will I put arthritis gel on my toothbrush? Call my son by his dog's name? (I've already done that.) Forget to…uh? Sometimes I stumble on my path.

We seniors nervously make fun of our apprehensions regarding aging and are sometimes dismissed by our doctors because of our age. But we are also being encouraged to thumb our noses at this culture's fear of aging and head into it with a self-embracing attitude, and a new set of longevity (and levity) tools. This book offers you tools.

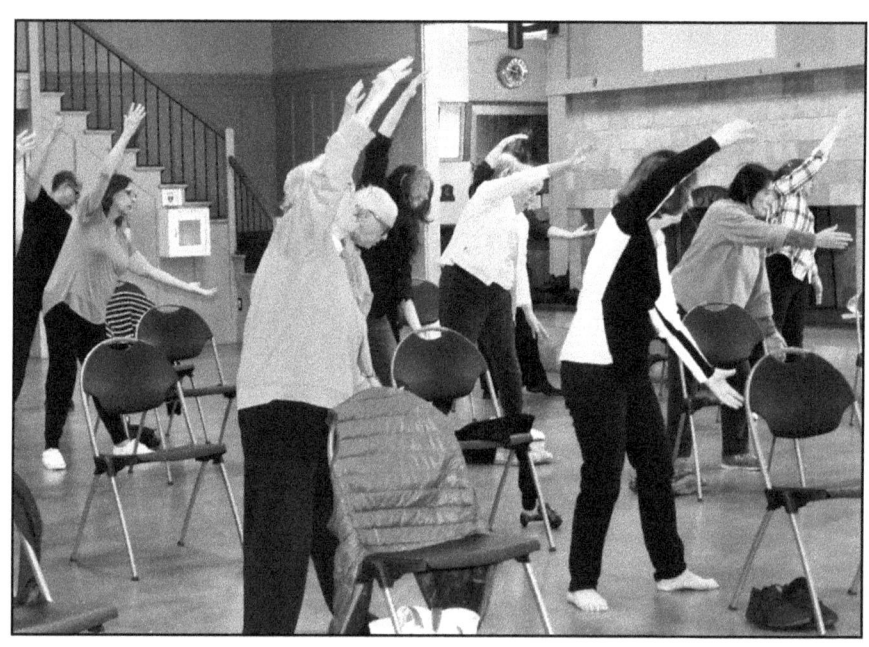

I

What Do We Mean By Balance?

*"Each of us is a conglomeration of a vast system...
Any influence on any aspect of the system will
affect every other aspect."*

T.K.V Desikachar

Balance is at the center of everything that exists in the ever-changing play of diverse forces. Balance, according to western mind/body science, is achieved through a complex process involving the interaction and coordination of several body systems and subsystems: the musculoskeletal system, sensory systems, and central nervous system. From this perspective, balance is defined as one's ability to maintain the body's center of gravity over the base of support whether stationary or moving.

According to the Eastern traditions, balance depends on the interplay of subtle life force energy (known in respective traditions as Qi, Chi, Ki, or Prana) in the physical, mental/emotional, and spiritual body. This energetic interplay is enhanced by relaxation in our physical body and mind. Throughout this book we will refer to the important role relaxation plays in preventing physical and mental rigidity, both hazardous to balance.

The etymology of the word 'balance' beginning in the 13th century comes from the Latin word 'bilanx', meaning two-sided pan or scale used in measure. During the 15th to 19th centuries, this definition of balance came to include a larger context of harmonious life balance with which we are familiar today.

In Asia balance is often depicted by the yin-yang symbol, representing the essential dance of diverse forces as inseparable parts of the whole. In this book, balance refers to all of the above: physiological, energetic, mind, body, and spirit and how that balance applies to an integrated mindful movement practice.

As mentioned in the introduction, there are some medical conditions that contribute directly to issues with balance that are outside the scope of this book and should be addressed by a medical professional (see page 10). It also goes without saying that adopting healthy life habits such as eating well, staying hydrated, getting enough sleep, avoiding poor footwear, maintaining positive social connection, and making sure our environment is supportive and well lit, all contribute to overall balance, and a reduced risk for falls in seniors.

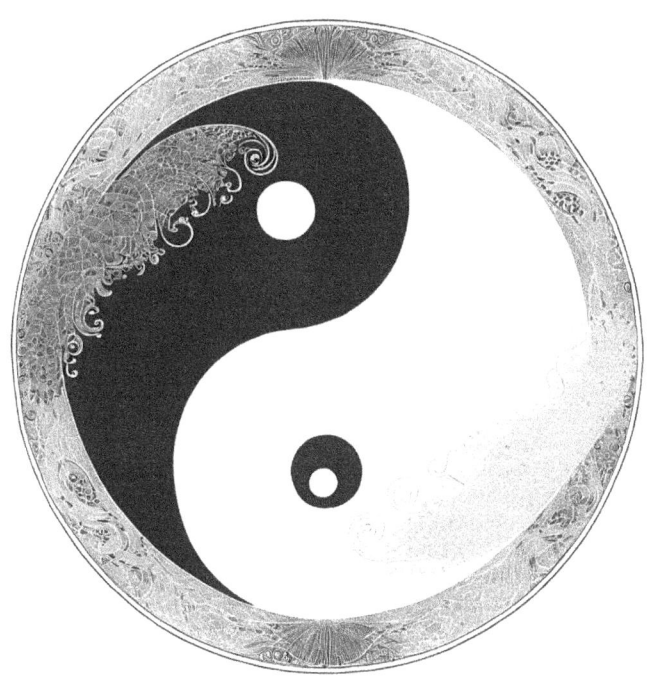

Medical conditions that may contribute to balance issues for seniors:

- Inner ear disorders and inflammation
- Psychiatric disorders such as anxiety and depression
- Heart disease
- Low or high blood pressure
- Thyroid disease
- Neurological disease: i.e. Parkinson's, Alzheimer's
- Stroke
- Anemia
- Diabetes
- Peripheral neuropathy
- Migraines
- Certain medications
- Uncorrected vision problems
- Head injury

   This is not a complete list

Other common factors that can increase risk of falls for seniors:

- Inadequate lighting
- Lack of handrails (stairs/bathrooms)
- Loose rugs
- Slippery or wet floors
- Split level floors
- Hazards (i.e. raised thresholds, clutter)
- Poor hydration
- Poor nutrition
- Lack of sleep
- Unsupportive footwear (i.e. high heels, overly stiff shoes)
- Alcohol or drugs that alter cognition

II

The Body Systems: 'Changes As We Age' and 'What We Can Do'

"When you adjust the posture and move the body gently, you balance and harmonize the internal water throughout the matrix... This internal array of rivers and oceans is propelled and circulated when you deepen the breath, when you contract the muscles, when you relax."

Roger Jahnke, O.M.D.

As we age the body naturally goes through changes that often have an adverse effect on balance, but we do not have to be at the mercy of these changes. We can improve our sense of stability and equilibrium, bring awareness to our vulnerabilities, and learn to trust our body and choices to serve us. With effort, our bodies are capable of gaining and retaining strength and flexibility well into our elder years.

The aging process is vastly different for everyone, as is our own make-up and circumstances. However, there are some common age-related changes to the systems of the body directly affecting balance. Western medicine is well versed in the general benefit of exercise for circulation, digestion, mood, and general well being. More specifically, we will describe in this section changes in the musculoskeletal system, sensory systems, central nervous system, and subtle energy system. Not everyone will experience all of these changes in significant ways. Keep in mind all systems are constantly working in tandem with each other. Any influence on one system of the body/mind will affect the whole.

Many fitness therapies emphasize the idea of "core strength," focusing on the musculoskeletal system as a support structure for the body. Research has pointed to four essential components of any fall-prevention training: muscle strength training, reaction training, balance training, and proprioceptive training. Yet, physiologically, our core also consists of the organs and breath. The musculoskeletal system depends on this innermost layer for fuel, just as the other systems depend upon the health of our musculoskeletal system.

Skin, which separates us from the outside world, is considered the most superficial layer of the body, and yet it contains nerve fibers that innervate our core. All these layers are connected by fascia (connective tissue) and lymph. The balance strategies in the Seniors in Balance program engage the deep, middle, and superficial structures of the body, establishing a multi-layered approach to cultivating true strength. All of the strategies work synergistically — with awareness, movement, breath, and energy underlying all of the body systems that affect balance.

The body itself is miraculous and mysterious in so many ways. You do not need to know the information in this book to benefit from the practices themselves. For those with curious minds, it is a step in understanding. The real knowledge, however, lies within.

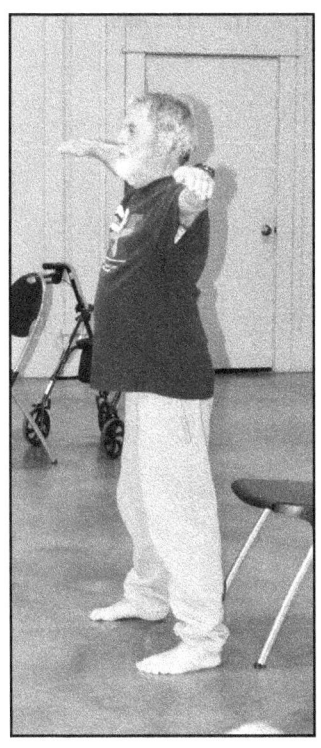

Shirley: Oh My Gosh

About 20 years ago, we were on our family vacation to the Sierras. Hiking to a favorite mountain lake, we came to a familiar log spanning a wide creek. Confidently, I started across the log, then froze. Oh my gosh — what's going on? I'd walked this log countless times, but this time I was shocked to find I was afraid I'd lose my balance. Now, in my 90s, thanks to the balance work, I walk confidently (though not on logs) and often, and enjoy a healthy active life.

Karen: Playing with Balance

As most children do, I remember feeling the joy of challenging my balance, hopping from boulder to boulder, or walking a beam. Children don't yet know all they are capable of, so they push themselves to see, repeating the task over again and gaining confidence.

Most older adults, as in Shirley's example above, eventually face a balance task that erases that confidence. Out of precaution they avoid situations altogether that challenge their balance.

Now, entering my senior years, I try to remember that childlike element of play, and attention to the way I walk on the earth throughout my day within a zone of safety.

Everyone can intentionally play with the vibrancy of their feet as they walk — notice the surfaces they walk on, and the connection they feel between their feet and the earth; pay attention to rolling through their feet, one continuous motion, like a wheel moving forward.

I like to walk on my tiptoes and then my heels, follow my son as he walks backwards up the hill, and practice walking on a small low-to-the-ground balance beam (this is not for everyone). I don't yet know what it will be like for me in my elder years, but I do know that in doing these things I already feel more aware, playful, and buoyant in my step.

Walking on cobblestones (and thus activating acupressure points in the soles of the feet), compared to regular walking, is shown by research to help improve balance, mobility, and blood pressure. It also positively affects mood.

It is important to remember (and practice using the muscles and nerve connections that help us) to not drop our toes as we walk. Walking heel to toe and pushing off with the toes is a wonderful exercise. It strengthens and enlivens the feet and ankles; helps maintain stability; engages the legs, pelvis, and spine; and is a great exercise for weight shifting and balance. It also keeps us from tripping over our own two feet.

The Musculoskeletal System

Calling to mind the musculoskeletal system, most of us tend to think first of strength and flexibility. Many seniors fear not being able to get up off the floor. This is primarily a function of strength and flexibility, along with proper positioning and focus. Clearly strength and flexibility are essential components of balance. But the role of the musculoskeletal system is more complex.

The musculoskeletal system controls your body's alignment, position in space, and motor activity. It also constantly communicates with your organs through biochemical signaling; is involved in processing glucose and regulating blood sugar (critical for healthy aging and cognitive function); interacts with your immune system to fight infection; helps you synthesize protein and metabolize amino acids; and affects your gut microbiome. Loss of muscle, common with aging, has been correlated in studies with a decrease in immune function and ability to fight infection. Increases in blood sugar, regulated by the health of the musculoskeletal system, directly impact brain function and nutrient absorption, which influences balance.

Your musculoskeletal system includes your bones, muscles, ligaments, tendons, and a large matrix of connective tissue called fascia. Your fascia runs throughout the body in deep (surrounding muscles, bones, nerves, and blood vessels), visceral (surrounding the organs) and superficial layers (just below the skin) of the body. It is a three-dimensional matrix made up of collagen proteins, immune cells and signaling molecules; and it helps stabilize the body. Without it we would not be able to stand upright. Fascia can over time and through injury dehydrate, tighten, and develop knots. Often, restriction we feel in our mobility and correlating pain in our body comes from compromised fascia. Releasing fascial restrictions can often relieve chronic pain, even in areas farther from the area of release.

Working in a physical therapy center many years ago, I (Karen) was introduced to a bodywork practice called Myofascial Release Technique™. It gave many of the patients experiencing chronic back pain more than just temporary relief. One concept in qigong is that the slow flowing movements help the fascia become more pliable and lubricated, and facilitate the free flow of energy and fluids through the matrix.

Misalignment in our abdominal core and vertebral column, due to age-related changes or injury to the musculoskeletal system, can compromise circulation of blood and lymph; and the joints and muscles may not receive the lubrication they need to stay strong and supple. Our walking gait depends upon integrity and flexibility in our spine, trunk, and pelvis as well as on strength and flexibility in our feet and ankles. Due to loss of flexibility, it is common to see walking gait in older adults that is slower, wider, shorter and flat footed. Many older adults, especially women, also lose bone density and mass, making fractures from falls more likely and serious.

The legs (particularly single leg standing and sit-to-stand capacity), feet, and ankles have to-date been the primary focus of most research and rehabilitation when it comes to improving balance in seniors. Studies have shown that in the foot and ankles, ankle flexibility, plantar sensitivity, and toe plantar flexor strength are significant factors in fall risks for seniors.

While not yet supported by clinical research and generally not addressed in balance training, recent literature and observational evidence suggests the arms, and particularly arm abductors (activated by raising the arms from the sides), play a significant role in maintaining balance during a sideways slip. Sideways falls are commonly responsible for fractures of the hip.

What We Can Do

Full Body Training

As we age, we need more full body training to keep our muscles strong and our fascia pliable, in addition to needing adequate protein intake to provide the building blocks to maintain and gain muscle mass. Using whole body movements, we engage in training the body to react, establish our alignment over our center of gravity, and focus our awareness on returning to that aligned stable center as we move.

Strengthening Core Muscles

The movements and forms in Seniors in Balance are designed to gently strengthen the core and stabilizing muscles upon which balance depends. We use the word 'gently' not to minimize the muscle strengthening components of practice but to emphasize the suitability and adaptability for seniors of any age, and the power of moving fluidly with awareness and varied intensity.

Head to Toe Movement

We awaken and strengthen the whole body, head to toe — engaging our feet, ankles, and legs as our foundation; our pelvic, gluteal (buttocks), and abdominal muscles in our core; our thoracic spine, chest, and neck in the upper body; and our arms and wrists. We also work with creating flexibility in the muscles and joints, lubricating the fascia and building a sense of spaciousness and alignment through our spine.

Lower Body Strength and Flexibility

Leg strength (peak muscle force) and power (strength plus contraction speed) are key components in all balance training, with sit-to-stand (STS) capacity (muscle power) being a key predictor of falls. We specifically practice sit-to-stand movement in a gradual sequence — activating the stabilizing muscles of the body and positioning ourselves over the center of gravity as we stand. In lower body training, we include strengthening the ankle dorsi flexor muscles (used in raising the foot and ankle — important for walking without tripping), knee flexors and extensors (used in straightening and bending the knee — important for knee stability), hip abductors (used when moving the leg away from the midline — important for weight shifting), and single leg strength, all critical for maintaining your balance.

Warming and softening the Fascia

Some movements warm and soften the facial tissue, allowing energy to flow more freely through the matrix of the body. The gentle rounded movements in Tai Chi/Qigong are beneficial for this, as well as the shaking (rebounding) movements and slow conscious release stretches.

Arm Strength and Flexibility

We improve arm abductor (moving the arm away from the body midline) strength and power of the arms by repeatedly raising and lowering of the arms, and swinging the arms throughout the movement sequence.

Weight Shifting

We also directly challenge static and mobile balance, focusing on shifting our weight to one leg at a time, shifting our weight back and forth, and doing single leg standing along with sit-to-stand exercises.

We learn to move 'smarter,' with less effort and more synergistically with body, breath, and awareness in sync.

The Neurological (Nervous) System

"Attend to the skin as a subtle boundary containing vastness. Enter that vastness and know there is no other but you."
Loraine Roche, PHD

Your balance depends upon proper functioning of your neurological system, carrying signals to and from your brain and body. Your balance works through a constant relay of information back and forth about your body's position in space and its conscious and unconscious adjustments. As we age, we may experience slower reflexes, slower nerve conduction, and decreased sensation in the peripheral nerves.

Our nervous system is divided into two main branches: the **central nervous system (CNS)** that carries signals to and from our brain through the spinal cord, and the **peripheral nervous system (PNS)** that refers to nerves throughout the body. The peripheral nervous system is divided into two subdivisions: the somatic nervous system and the autonomic nervous system.

The **somatic nervous system,** as discussed in the section above, carries sensory signals from your body to the CNS, and motor signals from your CNS to skeletal muscles to control movement in your body. It is considered voluntary, and within your conscious control.

The **autonomous nervous system** regulates internal physical processes such as heart rate, blood pressure, respiration, and digestion. It is considered largely (though not entirely), outside our conscious control. Breath is one important way we can consciously influence the autonomic nervous system. The autonomic nervous system is made up of elements of the brainstem, and some cranial and spinal nerves. It is further divided into *sympathetic, parasympathetic*, and *enteric* nerve fibers.

The **sympathetic branch** generally increases energy and govern the body's "fight or flight response." As we age, the sympathetic nervous system tends to become more dominant. The **parasympathetic branch** generally conserves energy and governs the "rest and digest" response. Of great importance is the vagus nerve, which means 'wandering nerve' in Latin, and is an important part of the parasympathetic nervous system. The vagus nerve is the longest of the 12 cranial nerves, and runs from the brainstem all the way into the abdomen. It innervates the throat, circulation, respiration, and digestion. It also activates the body's relaxation response, which is essential for health and balance. Vagal tone can decrease with age and a lifestyle of chronic stress, but it can also be consciously improved as with many of the flowing movement, breath, and energy practices offered in this book.

The **enteric system,** sometimes referred to as a "second brain," refers to a group of neurons in the gut wall that controls the gastrointestinal tract. Decrease in these neurons with age can affect motility. Gut health, directly related to overall well being and brain health, can also affect balance.

Our **brain** and **memory** are a part of our neurological system. Although age-related decline in cognitive ability varies greatly among individuals, studies have shown that fluid intelligence is the aspect of cognition most likely to change. Fluid intelligence ("native mental ability") refers to our information processing system. Our fluid intelligence is involved when we have trouble with the speed at which we analyze information (processing speed), difficulty discerning what is necessary for a task due to difficulty focusing (attention), or difficulty taking in new information from the environment or accessing memory stores (memory capacity).

When we experience a decline in fluid intelligence, it can affect our ability to integrate sensory cues from our environment, and slow our reaction times, thus affecting how our body responds to changes within and around us and our capacity to maintain balance.

Fluid intelligence is affected by both the cerebellum and corpus collosum areas of the brain. The cerebellum (back of the brain) is the part of the brain largely responsible for balance, muscle control, coordination, and eye movement. Basically, each hemisphere of the brain, left and right, sends signals to the cerebellum which coordinates and fine tunes those signals for motor control. The corpus callosum (the main pathway of nerves connecting the left and right hemispheres of the brain), also important for balance, delivers messages from one half of the brain to the other. As we age, both the cerebellum and corpus callosum commonly undergo a decline in size and function affecting motor skills, dexterity, gait, stability, and balance.

What We Can Do

Research has shown the good news that as we age our brains often become more densely wired on account of acquired learning and experience, and less rigidly bifurcated — meaning we have a greater capacity to use both hemispheres of the brain for a given task (crystallized intelligence). So, while our mind may not be as quick as in our youth, we are in fact generally wiser, and capable of making more balanced choices.

Boosting Brain Function

Research has identified physical exercise, challenging mental activities, achieving a "sense of control" or mastery, and social networking as the most effective ways to boost functioning of the aging brain. Barring pathology, our brain can continue to create neural pathways throughout our lifetime, as long as we give it the kind of exercise that stimulates neurogenesis (the creation of new neural pathways).

Karen: A Fall

It was an avoidable fall that landed my mother-in-law in the hospital with a fracture that never fully healed. She lived the duration of her life bedridden and on painkillers. This outcome is unfortunately not an uncommon story.

She had been a lively senior, full of enthusiasm, and lived a good long life. If I am lucky, my mind will remain as sharp as hers was late in her 80s. However, as someone who has deeply studied the body, movement, and healing, I was well aware that her gait was noticeably short and flat footed, with a significant curvature in the spine. She went from 5'2" tall to 4'8" in her elder years. Although she occasionally went for walks, she did not exercise regularly, and generally lived more in her head than body.

I wonder how might she have benefitted from the kinds of practices that would have strengthened her core and legs, improved circulation, and engaged awareness of her body and surroundings? Could she then have rebalanced when off kilter, broken her fall, noticed the obstacle on the ground to avoid tripping? Or sat down, breathed, and taken her time if she was dizzy?

Research shows that we can improve our balance with practice, and reduce our risk for falls. Making that kind of effort must always be a personal choice — something we want to do for ourselves. For those who do it is meant to be an enjoyable, adventurous, and nourishing endeavor.

Imagery

Along these lines, fluid intelligence is shown to correlate with the right frontal lobes of the brain stimulated by spatial awareness, imagery, and holistic thinking so often used in the Eastern-inspired and somatic movement practices as well as in the Seniors in Balance program. Positive visual imagery, an integral component of Qigong, can increase the neurotransmitters dopamine and seratonin in the brain, both important for memory function and mood.

Cross Lateral Movement

Seniors in Balance uses shaking and side-to-side movements as well as other appropriately mentally challenging movements that require coordination and integration of the left and right sides of the body. The cross-lateral movements we use in Seniors in Balance deliberately move the head and torso across the midline of the body, activating the brain across the corpus callosum.

Shaking and Bouncing

Research has shown rebounding exercises (such as on a trampoline) can increase blood flow to the brain and stimulate the vestibular and proprioceptive senses. A gentler form of bouncing, with a similar effect and more appropriate for seniors, is a Qigong rhythmic shaking movement that we incorporate in the Seniors in Balance program. Although a very simple movement, it consciously engages a sense of freedom or release of held stress in the joints and muscles (parasympathetic rest and digest response), and it promotes energy flow through the body. A neuroscientist and cranial sacral practitioner once told me that shaking and bouncing are akin to a nervous system reset, recalibrating the stress response.

Engaging the Eyes

When we connect the movement of our eyes (and other senses) with our awareness of the body, we stimulate the muscles, nerves, and tissues of the eyes (and the vagus nerve) intricately connected not only with the brain but also with the rest of the body. By engaging these connections and consciously using our eyes, we increase the communication pathways throughout our body, nervous system, and brain.

In the Seniors in Balance program we bring attention to our gaze and where we are focused, practicing looking near and far, and taking in the sensory cues around us as we are moving (see section on the sensory systems). It is common in Qigong and Tai Chi for the gaze of the eyes to follow the movement of the hands. This engagement of the eyes expands our visual field, engages our parasympathetic nervous system, and encourages mindful awareness. It is also common in Qigong to have the eyes open but soft, sending a message to the nervous system to be engaged but relaxed.

Activating the hands and Feet

Many nerve endings with important functions run throughout the hands and feet. In both yoga and Qigong hand gestures are an important aspect of many practices, facilitating the flow of sensory information and energy through the body/mind. Bringing awareness to our feet is also important. I noticed watching one of my students in class doing a balancing pose, that her balance had greatly improved. She said it was due to increased awareness or her feet and practicing rolling through her feet when walking.

Relaxation

Exercise itself helps regulate our metabolism which directly affects the functioning of our mood, brain, and nervous system. Deep breathing techniques, movement of the eyes, self-massage, somatic movement, chanting, organ sounds, mindfulness, and meditation all help tone the vagus nerve, relax the body/mind, and engage deeper awareness.

Karen: Chanting 'OM' (AUM) and Meditation

I have always loved the chant 'om.' According to ancient yogic texts, 'om' represents the primordial sound of creation, the origin seed (Bija) of all other sounds. Some texts even suggest it represents the purest base of life and of everything that exists.

Chanting 'om' also has a profound effect on the nervous system. Physiologically it de-activates the limbic (overactive during stress) part of the brain, inducing relaxation and focus. It activates the laryngeal muscles surrounding the vocal cords and lengthens the exhale, thus stimulating the vagus nerve and a parasympathetic relaxation response.

Chanting is a form of meditation. When we think of meditation, we often imagine someone sitting cross-legged on the ground. While that may be one form in which a meditation technique (quieting and focusing the mind) is practiced, meditation itself is a state of conscious absorption in the present (where there is no separation between the inner and outer consciousness).

There are many types of meditative techniques across all cultures. However, meditation can be practiced doing anything, and a meditative state can be present at any time. Yoga, Tai Chi, and Qigong (as all movement can be) are forms of moving meditation.

How does meditation relate to balance? The practice of meditation is one path in helping us relax the mind and body, bringing us into greater equilibrium and improving our entire mind/body connection. It can improve heart rate variability inducing a greater sense of calm and physiological balance.

The Sensory Systems

Our senses connect us with the outside world. They provide input via electrical signals through the nervous system to the brain regarding changes in our environment. These signals are essential for the body to regulate balance. In addition, our capacity to centrally integrate multi-sensory information (sensory integration) in the brain from the visual, vestibular, proprioceptive, and somatosensory systems is critical for balance control.

The sensory system includes both **general somatic senses** (receptors found all over the body — touch, pressure, temperature, position, vibration, and pain) and **special senses** (receptors found in specialized organs — visual, auditory/hearing, olfactory/smell, gustatory/taste, and vestibular/balance). Special senses send information to the brain via cranial nerves, while the general somatic senses send signals from the periphery of the body through the spinal cord to the brain.

While all of the special senses may affect overall balance in the body, we focus here on the **special senses** most directly known to impact balance in seniors: visual, vestibular, and auditory.

The visual system includes visual acuity, depth perception, contrast sensitivity, and peripheral vision. It tells us about the surface we are walking on and where we are in relation to what surrounds us. It is important to note that over 80% of our vision comes from the processing of visual information in the brain, rather than in the eyes. Much of the reduction in visual function that occurs with age is due to anatomical changes in the eyes such as decreased elasticity of the lens, weakening of the muscles surrounding the lens, and increased variations in the eyeball. These changes reduce the quality of sensory input we receive, making it difficult to navigate uneven surfaces and stairs; focus at close range; adapt to variable lighting conditions; and recognize objects and distinguish their edges, depth, and relative distance.

Visual acuity (the clarity or sharpness of vision); *contrast sensitivity* (the ability to distinguish between light levels on static image); *depth perception/stereo acuity* (the ability to see objects in three dimensions); *glare sensitivity; visual field size;* and *visual motion perception* have all been shown to contribute to our ability to maintain balance and reduce the risk of falls.

The auditory system, part of the inner ear along with the vestibular system, refers to the cochlea — the fluid-filled, spiral-shaped cavity where sound waves are changed into electrical impulses and transmitted to the brain. The auditory system shares with the vestibular system a nerve pathway to the brain (the vestibulocochlear nerve). Though they operate separately, they can impact one another. As with vision, over 80% of our 'hearing' comes from the processing of auditory information in the brain. When hearing declines with age, a lower quality of auditory cues is transmitted to the brain.

The vestibular sense involves hair cells in the inner ear that sense head position, head movement, and whether the body is in motion. Independent from visual clues, it provides information about up and down, side-to-side, and circling head movements in space, and also provides information about the speed and direction of movement.

Compensation that helps maintain balance involves three vestibular reflexes. The *vestibuloocular* reflex *(VOR)* modulates extrinsic eye muscles to maintain gaze during head movements; the *vestibulocollic reflex (VCR)* controls the neck muscles to stabilize the head's position in space during body movement; and the *vestibulospinal* reflex (VSR) controls the body and limb muscles to maintain posture and balance.

The vestibular system works closely with the visual and auditory system and plays a large role in maintaining balance; however, current research on age-related changes in the vestibular system is not conclusive. While hearing loss does not necessarily go hand in hand with a decrease in vestibular function, it can result in reduced quality of auditory cues, increased cognitive load, and increased sense of isolation — all capable of affecting balance. Sound can act as a kind of ballast, much like a focal point does for the visual system.

Changes in the vestibular system are thought to occur gradually over time, and partially in both ears. Reduction or loss of bilateral vestibular function results in difficulty maintaining balance especially when walking in the dark or on uneven surfaces, and a decrease in one's ability to see clearly while the head is moving. Loss of vestibular hair receptor cells in the inner ear and reduced ability for compensation by the vestibulor reflexes can also affect balance.

The terms equilibrium and postural sway are often used by doctors or physical therapists in evaluating someone's balance. *Equilibrium* is the coordination of movement strategies to stabilize the body's center, and maintain upright.

Postural sway refers to the constant subconscious small movements that happen around the body's center of gravity while standing still or moving to adapt to changes in our environment and maintain balance and stability. Postural sway involves the interplay between the musculoskeletal and sensory systems. The better the balance, the less postural sway.

The **general somatic senses** involve three subsystems: *exteroception* (detecting stimuli from outside the body), *interoception* (providing information about internal states), and *proprioception* (awareness of the position and movement of the body and head also known as kinesthesis). When changes in the environment are detected by the somato-sensory receptors, our body works to reduce the sensation and bring the body back into balance.

Exteroception involves sensory receptors responsible for detecting environmental changes on the body, primarily on our skin (tactile), such as pressure, vibration, and temperature.

Aging is accompanied by a steady decline in touch sensitivity and acuity, which can affect the capacity to detect when an object has come in contact with the skin. With age, there is often an overall decrease in the number of nerve fibers in the top and middle layers of the skin, as well as a decrease in the speed at which nerve signals travel. Although research shows that touch sensitivity declines, for some (not yet known) reason, gentle touch tends to become more pleasant as we age.

Interoception is responsible for providing information on internal states within our body such as the urge to urinate, hydration, the heartbeat, hunger, temperature, pain, and emotions. Interoception helps us maintain a state of homeostasis, is essential for our survival, and helps us maintain postural control. It has gained more attention in recent years as it has been shown to largely affect our ability to manage emotions and social interactions.

Interoceptive accuracy (the ability to detect internal changes) tends to decline with age. Lower interoceptive sensitivity has been shown to correlate with lower cognition and arousal. Practicing directing our awareness to internal cues can improve our interoceptive capacity.

Proprioception, a key component of balance for seniors, is responsible for detecting changes in our body's position and movement of the limbs and head in space. It is mediated by receptors encased in connective tissue in the muscles, joints, and ligaments. Proprioception allows us to walk without having to look at the ground. Proprioceptors of the ankles, knees, and cervical areas have been shown in studies to be important components in maintaining balance.

With age, the density of sensory receptors in our connective tissue, muscles, and superficial layers of the skin also tends to diminish, raising the threshold at which our body senses and responds to environmental changes. This decline in proprioceptive function can affect motor performance, including both reaction time and accuracy of motor responses, and increase postural sway (an important measure of balance).

Age may affect our capacity to centrally integrate sensory information from the visual, vestibular, proprioceptive, and somatosensory systems (sensory integration), which is important for balance control. Aging tends to slow the process of sensory re-weighting (the ability to adjust sensory information), suppressing erroneous sensory cues and becoming more sensitive to reliable ones. This slowing of the re-weighting process consequently lengthens the time it takes for postural adaptation. When we tilt our head sideways or experience a sudden turn in an airplane, it takes the messages from our inner ear canal longer to bring us back into equilibrium. When the nervous system cannot readily compensate for these changes in the vestibular system, we get dizzy.

> *Please note there are medical conditions outside the scope of this book that can affect our sense of balance and make us dizzy. Anyone experiencing these symptoms should consult a doctor to determine the cause.*

What We Can Do

Engaging and Expanding the Visual Field

We can specifically engage the visual system as we follow the movement of our hands through space; activate our eye muscles to look side to side, up, down, and in circles; turn our head to look over our shoulder and play with expanding our field of awareness; intentionally bring awareness to what we see in our horizon; and feel somatically noticing how the movement of the head and body connect with the movement of eyes, and even the inner ears and rest of the body.

We bring awareness to our gaze and where we are focused, practicing looking near and far, and taking in the sensory cues around us as we are moving. It is common in Qigong and Tai Chi for the gaze of the eyes to follow the movement of the hands. This engagement of the eyes expands our visual field and engages our relaxation response. The common practice of softening the eyes in Qigong helps expand peripheral vision and awareness while also relaxing the eyes.

Challenging the Vestibular System

Eye movements, shoulder shrugs and circles, moving the head through space, weight shifting, and full body movements all challenge the vestibular system and help the brain recalibrate to improve balance.

Improving Proprioceptive Function

Muscle strengthening and balance exercises are shown to help improve proprioceptive function. Also bringing blood flow to the joints, particularly in the feet, ankles, knees, and in the cervical spine, may improve proprioception. Some studies have shown that older adults who did Tai Chi regularly, had better joint proprioception and balance control while weight shifting.

Stimulate the Skin

The tactile sense, mediated by sensory receptors located in the upper layers of the skin, is stimulated by self-massage practices.

Karen: Hearing and Listening

I recently had a baseline hearing test. The results were interesting. As the audiologist played various tones, I listened intently. When the hearing test was over, I confessed to the audiologist that I had no idea how many of the sounds I actually 'heard.' As the sounds became fainter and my ears alone could not pick up the tones, I still sensed they were there and pressed the button to register the sound.

The audiologist was non-plussed by my confession. He said it did not matter. I fared very well on the test. I wonder: How much does awareness and 'presence' govern the capacity of our senses?

Wearing hearing aids is known to reduce fall risks in those with hearing loss. It improves the quality of sensory input in those who need them. However, what we do with that information is in the brain and in our awareness.

One day in class, there was some very loud jack hammering going on in the room next door. Nobody could hear me and the sounds for the students were nerve-racking. I could see frustration in everyone's faces mounting. I stopped the class and suggested we move together in silence (see and feel without my talking). In a short while, the movements of everyone in class were beautifully in sync. The shift towards greater inner focus was clear.

They were feeling more fully into the movements and focusing on internal rather than external cues. Practicing with presence and 'deep listening' is a cornerstone of the Eastern-inspired movement arts, and an essential element of balance.

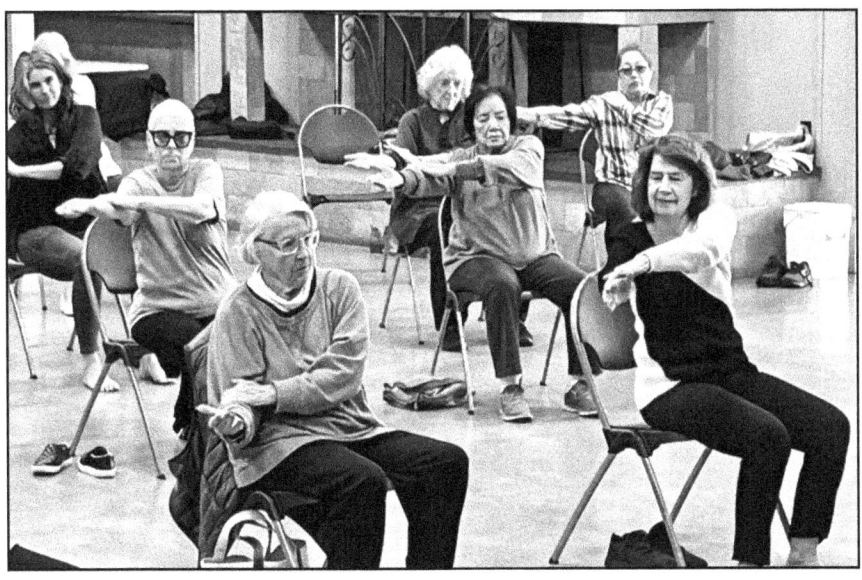

Subtle Energy System

"Like a cool breeze or the warmth of a fire, prana and Qi are perhaps more easily understood when felt and experienced."

Omega Institute

Intuitively, most of us know that maintaining a balanced flow of energy in our body/heart/mind is key to good health and well-being. While this philosophy has been around for ages, modern science is increasingly interested in studying the science behind it — a field of study called Biofield science. A Biofield is defined as a supposed field of energy or life force that surrounds or permeates a living thing. Researcher Jain Shanini, PhD, calls it "a new term by western scientists to describe some things we've known for a long time."

In Eastern traditions, invisible life force energy is referred to as **Prana** (in Ayurveda and yogic traditions), **Qi** (in Chinese medicine and Tai Chi/Qigong; also spelled 'Chi'), and **Ki** (in Japan). While science does not yet explain how it happens, research has shown that energy has intelligence that transfers over distance to affect health.

According to Qigong master Robert Peng, Qi is *"an invisible but discernible type of energy that permeates our bodies, much like an electromagnetic field, and powers our vital functions."* It also encompasses the spiritual energy "Shen." According to the ancient traditions, when energy flow is blocked, it can disrupt the vital and unified functioning of the body/mind/spirit, and eventually create imbalance in our body. Many people describe energy flow in the body as subtle energy. As Nobel Prize-winning scientist Albert Szert-Gyorgyi says, "Nature is simple but subtle."

The vast communication network of fascia is now considered a conduit for electron flow, which is essential for health. Fascial lines in the body correlate closely with the meridian system of Traditional Chinese Medicine (TMC) and Qigong, which may explain how working with those pathways works in supporting and balancing the body systems.

In yoga, breath and energy share the same word: 'Prana' (often referred to as primordial breath or life force energy). Breath is the most fundamental function of life from the moment we are born to the moment we die. It is also one of the few involuntary processes in the body that can be consciously controlled, and a primary way of working with the flow of subtle energy in the body.

Prana is also considered a powerful gateway of higher consciousness. Awareness of the breath and different types of breathwork can quiet and focus the mind, shift us out of a Beta brain wave state (active thinking), relax our body/mind, and help us become more present.

Research has shown that intention also has a profound effect on the energy field in the body and on healing. In our western culture, aging is often viewed as a loss of everything that gives meaning and importance to life. Yet in some cultures, where elders are revered as the apex of wisdom and compassion, the life force often stays strong. In his book *The Heart of the Hunter*, author Laurence Van Der Post says, *"Old is the most revered word in the Bushman language."*

If we have a negative attitude about aging, our body and psyche tend to oblige. If we hold on to grievances and grip against change, we may hold ourselves back from experiencing the wonder and wisdom of our elder years. We can instead focus our mind on our connection with the creative, life-giving force of the universe, and direct that energy through the channels of the body.

Traditional Chinese Medicine (TMC) theorizes that as we age, the energy reserves in the kidneys *(prenatal Qi)* diminish, compromising the vitality of the body. However, through conscious awareness, imagery, and energy practices we can cultivate the flow and strength of Qi *(acquired Qi)*, helping to keep our bodies and minds strong.

In the United States, where we live, our culture is, in general, inherently more yang (active) than yin (receptive), driven by the pursuit of external success and acknowledgement. With the constant demands of modern life, many people overwork and do not take time to replenish until it becomes a well-worn habit. As cultural anthropologist Angeles Arrien, and author/teacher of the Four-Fold way, used to say, "The pace of nature is medium to slow." In order to be in tune with our natural rhythm, we must take time to slow down, feel, listen, and receive. This is true also within a movement or balance practice. We come back repeatedly to our center.

As we age, it becomes more difficult to ignore the needs of our body, mind, and spirit, because our ability to compensate for these energetic imbalances decreases. Hence, to regularly bring balance and peace to our whole system is to nurture our life force.

What We Can Do

Balancing Renewal and Activity, Yin and Yang

As we embrace the natural changes of our aging body, we can enter into a deeper internal relationship with ourselves, and reconnect with the longing of our soul to express our authentic nature. Attending to the balance of building strength and energy, and taking time for nourishment and relaxation, is necessary for our health. We use imagery and internal awareness to direct the flow of energy through the body/mind, and connect with the world inside and around us.

We attend to the natural flow of breath through the body, connecting with the expanding, energizing energy of the inhale, and the grounding, calming energy of the exhale — breathing in synchronicity with our movement. We also connect with the larger breath of the Earth and universe bringing us in relationship with our larger presence.

Opening and Directing the Flow of Energy Through the Body

Many of the movements of Tai Chi/Qigong and yoga intentionally open energy pathways and gates in the body, and enliven the primary centers of energy (the three Dantiens in Qigong).

The slow, fluid movements of Tai Chi/Qigong, yoga, and other mind/body practices keep the rivers of subtle energy flowing: nourishing body, mind, spirit; replenishing our reservoirs; building strength; sharpening our senses; and calling forth the self-healing tendencies inherent in our human nature to create vitality, balance, and 'union.'

Relaxation

The most common comment we get from our students is that the class makes them feel so relaxed, while also strengthening their body. Relaxation is an important, and often overlooked, aspect of building strength and resilience. It is key to restoring and increasing the natural flow of energy in the body, reducing chronic stress that creates havoc on all of the body systems, and improving mental focus and natural awareness.

With an emphasis on integrating breath, movement, imagery, and awareness, relaxation comes naturally and we are able to bring greater balance and vitality to all systems of the body/mind, improve blood flow to the tissues, breathe more deeply, and be more present throughout the day.

One of my client's proclaimed she was unable to meditate, having tried and 'failed' on a number of occasions. We did a short, very simple breath awareness meditation. When asked how she felt afterwards, she said "more relaxed, more calm and centered" - one of the great gifts of meditation. It is often easier than we realize to find that center.

Shirley: The Tao (Dao)

"Go with the flow" is a common refrain we hear in modern life. What flow?

According to the Taoists, there is an undefinable, unending river of energy propelling all life. They call this the Tao, which means 'the way.' For me, the Tao feels like a beautiful dance of movement, vibration, and life.

III

The Contributions to Balance of Eastern Practices

"The body instinctively avoids all harsh and aggressive motion, dictated by pressure to 'fragmentary' movements; instead, it accepts rounded movements, born of the spine and therefore leading to 'total action'."

Vanda Scarvelli, *Awakening the Spine*

Some common questions we often get from students are: Why do I feel so much change in my body when the movements are so subtle? What is Qigong and how is it different from Tai Chi? How do yoga and Qigong improve my balance?

In order to get the most out of what yoga, Qigong and Tai Chi have to contribute to improved balance, it helps to have a fundamental understanding of each these practices. While we focus on these three well established traditions, we also want to acknowledge the many wisdom traditions around the world that contribute to our understanding of a broader view of health and balance.

Yoga, Qigong, and Tai Chi, in their many forms, ground and strengthen the body, flow with the breath, engage the senses, and clear and rewire the mind through visualization, imagery, and meditation. They bring our awareness to our internal experience and our connection with the larger environment and universe. The holistic practices help us forge new connections in our brain's pathways, relax into our deeper experience, and allow our innate healing capacities to manifest. The ultimate purpose is the awakened union of body, mind, and spirit.

According to ancient traditions there is an intricate and extensive network of energy channels that enlivens and balances our system. This network is well described in both Traditional Chinese Medicine (TCM) and the Indian medical science of Ayurveda, although each in their own way. These invisible rivers of energy traverse and irrigate the entire landscape of the body.

In each of these traditions, this landscape is composed of five elements. Although each offer a subjective map of energy in the body and differ in emphasis, they both remind us of our deeper connection with the energy, rhythms, and seasons of nature…and that health can come to us through balance in these forces.

Qigong (pronounced 'chee gong'), grandfather of the martial arts and Tai Chi, is a meditative healing movement art and ancient Eastern science, which originated in China more than 5,000 years ago. There are different styles of Qigong depending on its purpose (medical Qigong, spiritual Qigong, or martial art Qigong), and many different forms.

According to Qigong theory, human beings are a microcosm of the Earth and universe and mirror its cyclical energies. The universal energies ('Qi' or 'Chi') loop through us in a network of invisible rivers, or channels, called meridians. There are 12 primary meridians, each relating to an organ whose function it influences. Hence, they are referred to as organ meridians. Health depends upon the unobstructed and balanced flow of Qi through these meridians.

The Meridian System incorporates the concepts of yin and yang, the two complementary yet opposing forces of the universe that make up a unified whole. Yin flows inward towards the core, and downwards towards the earth. Yang radiates outward and upward. Balance depends upon the harmonious interplay of these opposing forces.

Along these meridians are places called gates where the flow of energy is more easily felt and influenced. In Qigong, there are three key *Dantiens* or energy storage centers. The first Dantien (vitality) is located just below the navel. The second Dantien (love) is at the heart. The third Dantien (wisdom) is in the middle of the head. Balance in these three centers is critical for a balanced and healthful life.

Qigong self-massage involves touching the skin along the location and direction of the gates and meridians, intentionally activating the flow of subtle energy through the body and organs.

"Gong" (in Qigong) means to work or cultivate. The practice of Qigong cultivates the flow of Qi through rhythmic waves of breath and fluid movements that mimic the flow (Tao) of nature. The repetitive quality of these movements cultivates strength, balance, and increased coordination among mind, breath, body, and spirit.

Biomedical Research on Qigong is limited, but it has been shown to reduce stress and have a cascade of health benefits such as: improved balance, strength, blood pressure, resting heart rate, and immune function; a reduction in anxiety and depression; and possibly a reduction in pain. From the millions of people who regularly practice Qigong in Asia, and now in the west, the practice is well known to promote healthy longevity, speed recovery, enhance mental clarity and emotional stability, and prevent and deter degenerative diseases.

Tai Chi (a form of Qigong that falls in the category of a martial art) includes practices beneficial to balance: one's deeply rooted connection with the earth, whole body movement, fluid movement, flexibility of the spine, and ability to transfer weight from side to side while maintaining balance. As one develops these skills in Tai Chi practice, one also improves one's stability, centeredness, and confidence. Forms of Tai chi and Qigong often share similar movements. Tai Chi, however, may involve more rooting in the legs for stability while sparring. Qigong tends to engage greater opening at the front of the body (important for so many of us with constricted chest and abdominal areas) which is considered a vulnerable position in martial arts.

Modern research suggests Tai Chi can lead to significant improvements in balance, cardio-respiratory fitness *(forced vital capacity and peak oxygen uptake)*, cognition *(global cognition and executive function)*, mobility, proprioception, sleep and strength, as well as significant reductions in the incidence of falls, non-fatal stroke, and reduction in stroke risk factors.

Tai Chi is often recommended to seniors as a way to improve balance. A study by the National Institute on Aging (NIA), which was published in the American Medical Association (AMA) journal in 1996, suggested that Tai Chi brings about a statistically significant decrease in the number of falls in elderly participants.

The Seniors in Balance program has selected Tai Chi/Qigong moves which counter age-related changes in balance. Many seniors drop out of Tai Chi because the movements are too difficult to execute, or the sequences too difficult to remember. Therefore, we incorporate simple Tai Chi/Qigong movements in our teaching which eliminate those obstacles yet retain the balance benefits.

We incorporate movements that are gently strengthening, simple, repetitive, and challenging enough but safe to execute for seniors, and yet share the benefits of more complex forms of Qigong and Tai Chi. The meditative aspects of Tai Chi/Qigong reduce the stress, excessive worrying, low energy, and fear of venturing out, which can often accompany aging.

Yoga dates back more than 4,000 years in India. Through time yoga has evolved into many branches, and the numbers and kinds of yoga practices are vast. The word 'yoga' means to 'join together' or 'yolk.' In essence, it is the practice of uniting aspects of the self — physical, energetic, mental/emotional, and spiritual in order to experience our natural state of being, or rather realize the union which already exists. Like Qigong, the practice of yoga cultivates strength, grounding, flexibility, relaxation, focus, and a balanced flow of energy through the body.

While the yoga of the west is often seen as primarily a physical practice, classical yoga is traditionally a more complete practice and involves yama (morality), niyama (self-inquiry), asana (yoga postures), pranayama (breath control), pratyahara (a "gathering towards" of the senses for introspection), dharana (focused concentration), dhyana (meditation) and samadhi (state of enlightenment//bliss), all of which affect our well-being.

Yoga therapy is a more recent field of study (dating back to the 1920s) that adapts the practice of classical yoga to address specific health challenges and populations — in this case to address balance in seniors. It is derived from the yoga tradition of Ayurveda, the traditional medical practice of India. As with Tai Chi/Qigong, both these ancient traditions view the body as a microcosm of the larger universe. Yoga and Ayurvedic philosophy identify a series of channels (nadis) through which universal life force energy (prana) flows. Blockages in this flow of subtle energy through the body affect the balance and health of the body/mind. Balance is nurtured through practices of postures (asanas), breath (pranayama), awareness, mudras (hand gestures), sound, guided imagery, meditation, and relaxation.

In Ayurveda the subtle energy body is made up of nadis (channels), chakras (gates or centers) and marmas (points). The word Nadi comes from the root "nad" which means movement or stream. It refers to the innumerable arteries of subtle energy running through the body. The three main nadis are the sushumna (central channel of the spine); the ida (down the left side of the spine); and the pingala (up the right side of the spine). Harmonizing and balancing these essential forces of energy is a key to good health.

Chakras are transforming energy centers located along the central channel of the spine. They relate to the five elements of earth, water, fire, air, and ether

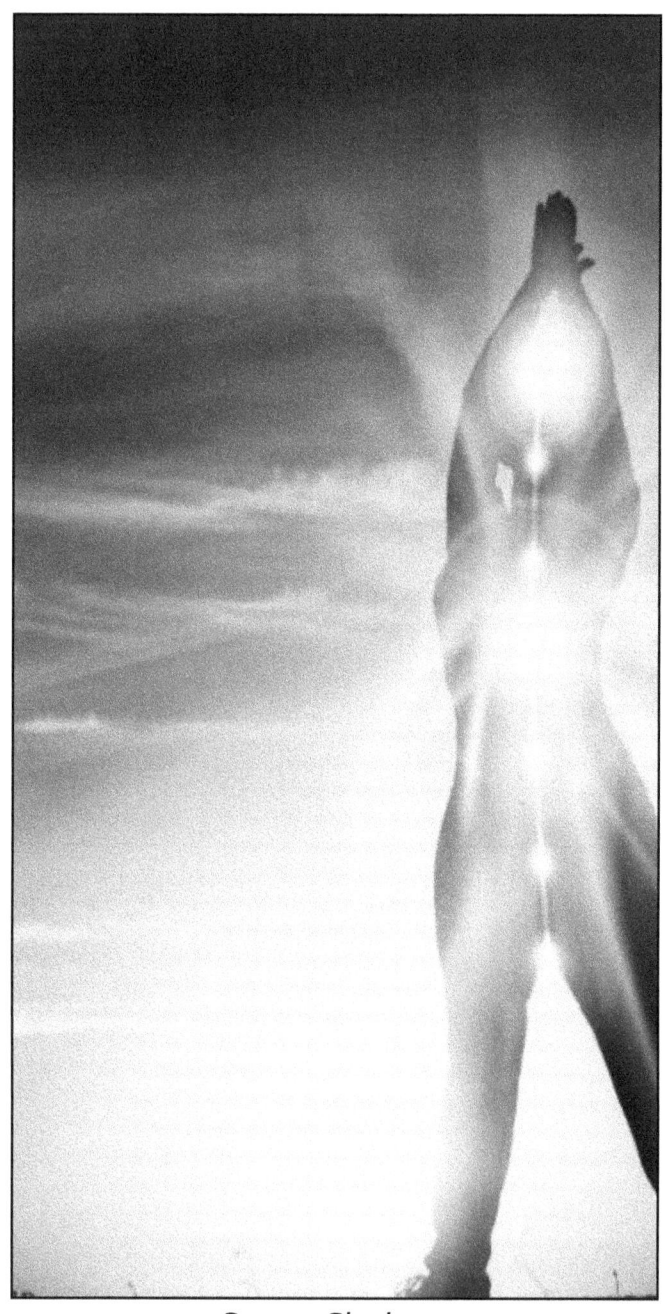

Seven Chakras

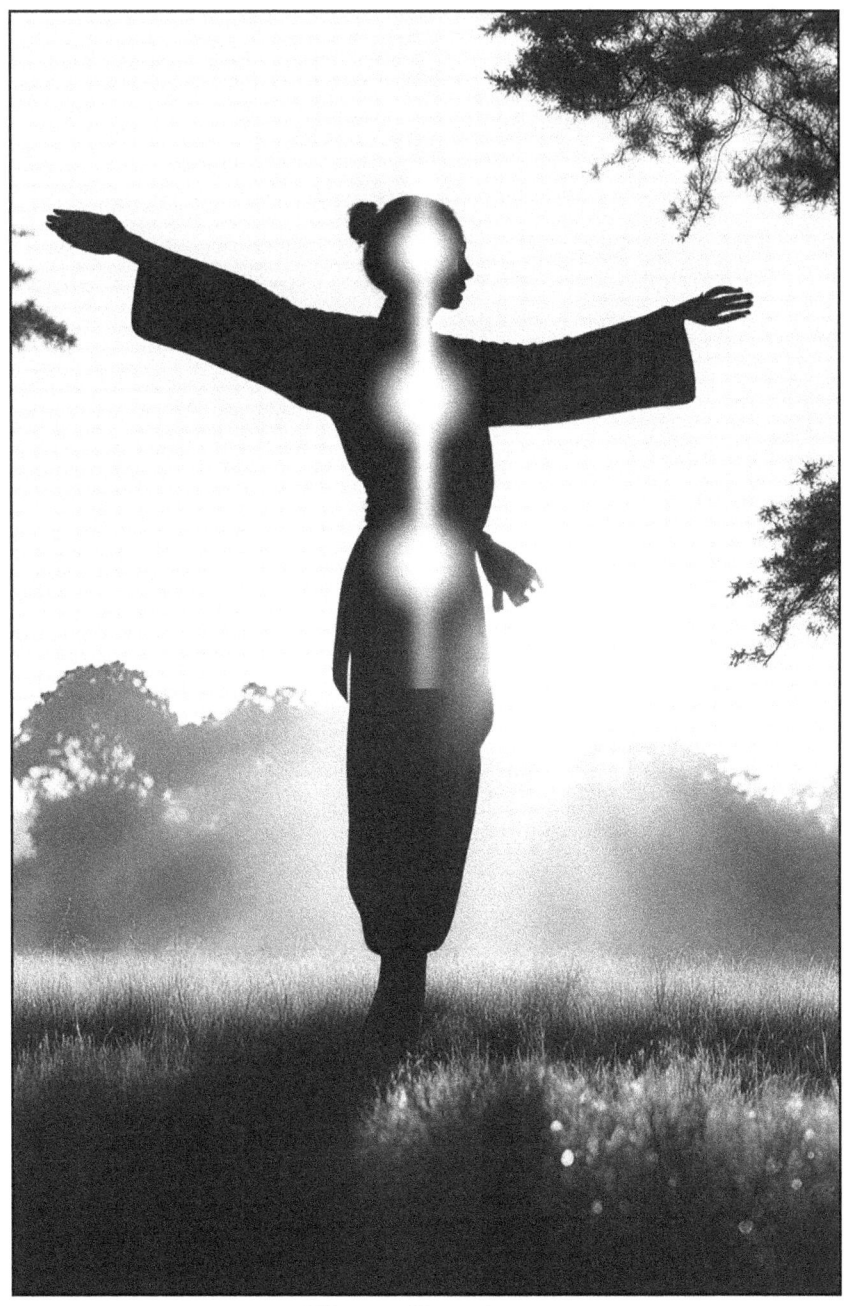
Three Dantiens

(space). They are considered energy centers or vortexes where physical, mental, subtle, and spiritual energies are linked and balanced.

Research has shown yoga has far-reaching health benefits. It is best known for its stress-reducing effects. Practiced appropriately, it has long been known to improve balance, strength, and flexibility in the musculoskeletal system; to increase circulation of blood, nutrients, and oxygen to the tissues and organs; to calm and balance the nervous system; to improve respiration and coordination; to balance the flow of energy through the body; and to focus and clear the mind.

A 2022 study by the National Institutes for Health states that yoga exercise intervention improves balance control and prevents falls in seniors. And that "a four-week yoga-based intervention had positive effects on static, dynamic, and total balance scores, body composition, and social status."

All yoga practices in this program are adapted to the senior population and for the purpose of enhancing a practice in balance. We incorporate postures, breath, meditation, sound, imagery, and relaxation, blending principles and practices of yoga and Tai Chi/Qigong. Some practices are done with the aid of a chair or seated; while all practices offer an option to sit.

IV

The Contributions to Balance of Western Mind/Body Methods

Modern Mind-Body Methods refer to training of the body/mind through harmonious integration of functional movement, mental focus, and controlled breathing to improve health. Unlike the origins of the Eastern traditions, these exercises are free of religious or spiritual influence.

Western mind/body exercise philosophy was first documented in the 1800s as part of gymnastics training. Although natural movement harmonizing exercise was likely a more ancient practice in the western world.

Toward the end of the 19th century, the regular use of holistic exercise training for gymnastics and sports shifted toward muscle building and weightlifting, leading to the culture of body building we see in gyms today.

Consequently, many of those who taught a holistic training approach branched out to create their own independent schools of thought. Most well-known among these are Frederick Matthias Alexander (1869-1955), who created The Alexander Method, and Joseph Hubertus Pilates (1880-1967), who created the Pilates Method. Multiple other methods have developed since, including the Feldenkrais Method. All of these pioneers used their functional integrative movement approach to effectively strengthen and heal their bodies from health challenges they encountered in their own lives.

In the 1960s, philosophy professor and movement theorist Dr. Thomas Hanna coined the term 'somatics' to refer to the body as perceived from within by first-person perception. "Soma" in ancient Greek means "living organism." Somatic movement approaches emphasize the cultivation of body awareness, relaxation of physical tension, and awakening natural movement patterns in the body.

Mindfulness programs, notably the Mindfulness Based Stress Reduction (MSBR) program, originally developed by Jon Kabat-Zin, has gained recognition in research and medical communities as an effective stress reduction tool. MSRB, although adapted for a secular western medical context, was founded on the principles and practices of eastern traditions, notably yoga and Buddhism. These programs have moved more and more mainstream and are finding their way into medical practice as the health benefits are profound.

Both slow functional movement and more active movement of strength and aerobic training have their benefits when it comes to aging and balance. What is emerging today is a more integrated perspective to health that incorporates mindful awareness, breath and energy flow, core strength building, flexibility, integrative/functional movement, and relaxation (coupled with some form of aerobic activity).

Some of the exercises in the Seniors in Balance program are derived from Pilates, Feldenkrais, and somatic-based movement training.

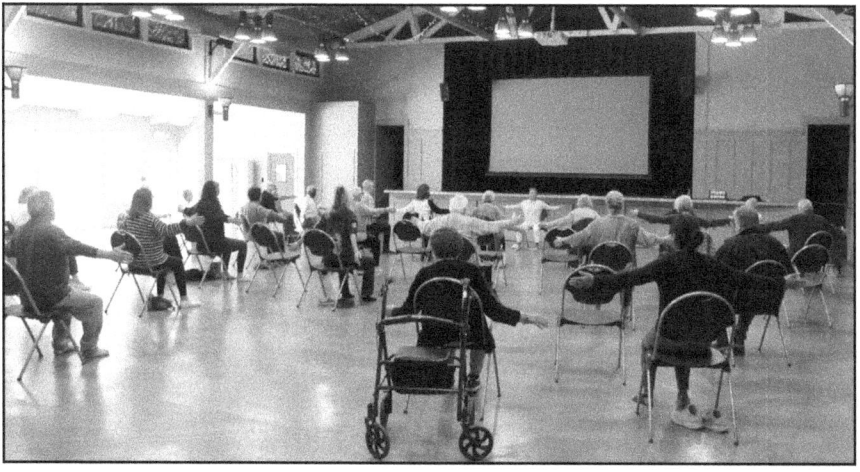

Karen: Limitation

As seniors, we have all experienced some sense of limitation in our body. If we try too hard to push past these limitations, we often make things worse. On the other hand, if we hold too tight, presuming that limitation is set in stone, we affirm a static state.

However, if we come to the edge of our limit (not over it), that is often where we do our best work. And what was once a limit is no longer.

We can apply this concept to so many things in life, not the least of which is building strength and balance in our bodies. In my own body, and in teaching others, I have seen how powerful subtle movement and energy practices can be in building health from the inside out. I have sometimes had students say it doesn't feel like they are working that hard in class but somehow they notice a big difference in their body.

We sometimes expect exercise to be hard work in order to gain momentum, feeling the need to 'push' through our limitations. Sometimes this is necessary, but long-term gain without repercussions is often made with more grace and listening step by step.

V

The Essence of Practice

"Healing can be understood as a movement towards dynamic balance, which brings us closer to our true essence. The intention to heal is a process of creating space for the natural wisdom of consciousness to guide us toward wholeness."

Jain Shanini, PhD

Like life, creating enduring strength, flexibility, self-assurance, and balance is not a linear process; it is a rich tapestry of experience. Each time you come upon a new thread there is an opportunity for growth and deep healing.

It is important to acknowledge how you feel when you begin a practice, and to listen to what your body needs. The more you become attuned to the subtle and not so subtle changes in your mind and body, and the effect your practices have on you, the more you are able to choose activities that nourish you and create better balance in all areas of your life.

Some qualities of mind that infuse the way one experiences a practice may seem quite obvious at first, and are true of life in general, but they deserve mention as it is often during a meditation or movement practice that one's long-held judgements, fears, and limiting beliefs arise and provide a rich opportunity for transformation.

Curiosity

Like any relationship, bringing a sense of curiosity to the adventure is what makes it fun and interesting. If you begin your practice with the mind of an explorer without a fixed agenda, it takes you back to a childlike state of wonder, and your emphasis shifts more to the present process than a pursuit or goal down the road.

Compassion

The heart is a receptive and generous organ. Allowing rather than forcing means your strength flows from your center and grows as you are ready. With compassion for yourself with all your limitations, along with gratitude for your strengths, you foster the patience to integrate your learning into everyday life.

Trust

An essential part of any practice is to trust in your body wisdom; in your capacity to heal (even if not always in the expected fashion); and in the depth of change that can come from leaning into that trust. The real gift of practice comes with relaxing into, trusting, and following the wisdom your body reveals.

Connection

Your body is a community of cells, fluids, connective tissue, energy, intelligence, and mystery. The more you re-discover your connection within as a wonderfully collaborative universe, the more you grow in depth, expansion, and connection in all realms of life. Connection within yourself, with others, and with the larger world all go hand in hand.

Intention

There will always be distractions: everyday noises from outside that command your attention, worries or agendas that run your thoughts amuck as you try to focus, or (for so many of us seniors) aches and pains that can consume your energy. The intent is not to ignore what is going on for you (by all means listen to your body), but to remind yourself that those distractions are just that and not the whole of you or your experience.

Creativity

While all the practices and traditions are a beautiful starting point for learning, it is in your unique expression, sense of joy, and how you relate to the practice and make it work for you, that makes it an art.

Breathe, breathe, breathe

Your conscious breath is your entryway into your wondrous body. When you breathe, you connect with the breath of the whole universe and also with the most fundamental, primordial function of your body from birth onward.

As author Peter Matthiessen states, *"In this very breath that we now take lies the secret that all great teachers try to tell us."*

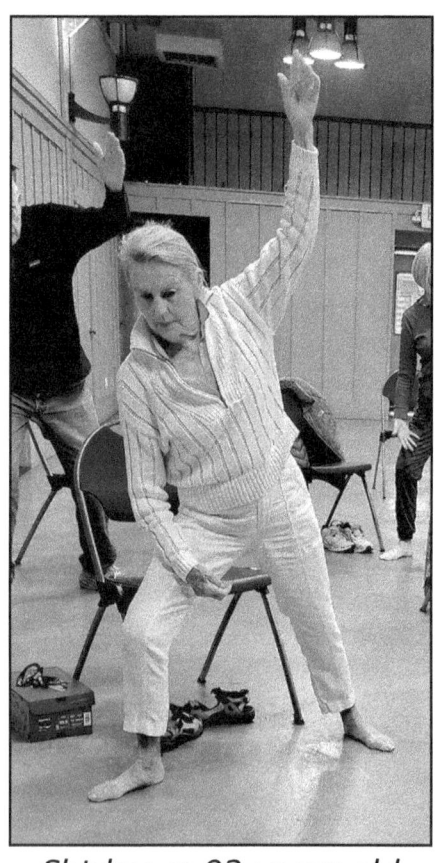

Shirley at 92 years old

Karen: The Blend of Forms

When I first began yoga, I was drawn to the grounding and strengthening elements it offers. It served me well at a time when I had a busy professional life and most needed that. As time has passed, I have come to appreciate and practice Qigong more and more, and love the sense of directed energetic flow and spaciousness the practice brings.

For Shirley, she fell in love with the fluid movements of Qigong, and for many years now Qigong has been her primary practice. However, as she has moved into her elder years, she has rediscovered how much she benefits from the warrior and other poses of yoga that ignite a sense of strength and grounding in her body and mind, and counterbalance the sense of frailty that comes with advanced age. If I teach a few classes in a row (which she now attends) where I leave out the yoga warrior poses, she asks if I can please bring them back because she misses them.

Together, yoga and Qigong complement each other well in terms of creating a well-balanced practice. It is when the movement practices (yoga, Qigong, Tai Chi) become a sort of dance (Tao) that they grace all movement, all stillness, all beingness throughout the day.

VI

The Structure of a Class or Personal Practice

"The human body is the universe in miniature. That which cannot be found in the body, is not to be found in the universe. Hence the philosopher's formula, that the universe within reflects the universe without. It follows that if our knowledge of our own body could be perfect, we would know the universe."

Mahatma Ghandi

While there are a variety of exercises that we may vary throughout any particular class or practice (and each practice can be practiced and explored on its own), there is an essential set of components we try to incorporate in a larger senior class: *preparation; grounding, centering, and establishing favorable alignment; fostering awareness; opening to the breath; warming up the body gradually for full-body movement; building strength and flexibility in the musculoskeletal system; quieting and focusing the mind; nourishing the body with energy.*

For seniors, we recommend moving into each exercise, pose, or stretch gradually in steps in order to bring attention to all components of the movement, and to enhance the feeling of safety within the movement. Movement can range for each person from a subtle small movement to something larger depending on what suits their needs. In a stretch it is important to move slowly; stop at the first barrier where you feel resistance; and wait for the tissue to warm, soften, and relax. When you feel a bit of release, you can move further allowing the stretch to unfold rather than forcing it. This helps gently soften and release the fascial tissue often contributing to stiffness in the senior population.

An important concept to keep in mind throughout your practice is to focus the mind, body, and breath on relaxation both in stillness and movement ('effortless engagement'). This is the way of creating true strength and natural energy flow within. Should you feel stress or tension build, adjust your posture, clear your mind, and deepen and relax with your exhaling breath.

Preparation

The beginning of a practice can be like standing at a gate. You take a moment, pause, relax, and stand present at the gate before opening. It is a moment of silence full of possibility, where we have yet to discover what our efforts will bring. When you don't take this moment to gather your attention and connect with your intention before you begin, you may take longer to show up fully for what you are doing.

Grounding, Centering, and Establishing Favorable Alignment

Balance begins with adjusting your posture and feeling connected with the earth and your body center. This means feeling your feet on the ground, bringing awareness to your center, feeling a lift through your crown at the top of the head, and creating space and alignment in the spine.

Grounding creates a sense of safety, stability, and support — with the feet, legs, and pelvis connecting you with the energy of the earth, the environment around you, and your physical reality. Grounding creates the foundation upon which you stand.

Centering connects you to your core in the abdomen, where the liberating, ascending energies (yang) and manifesting, descending energies (yin) meet. Energy also radiates from your central core to the periphery, and draws energy back from the periphery to your center.

Favorable alignment enables the free flow of energy, breath, and movement. Alignment is a dynamic process always adapting to the internal and external influences on your body over the base of support. As seniors, favorable alignment looks different for each of us. Some of us may have more curvature in the spine or other restrictions. Favorable alignment is done not with a goal of perfect posture. The focus is on the intention to bring yourself into a comfortable, relaxed but engaged, upright position, be it standing or sitting. You release held tension, and notice the subtle adjustments to posture that come with your awareness of breath. Balance is a dynamic state of constant micro and macro re-adjustment.

Opening to Breath

Movement and breath flow together rhythmically carrying life force through your body. When you bring your attention to your breath, it naturally tends to deepen. If you notice the pause at the beginning and end of the inhale and exhale, you can take a moment to enter this original stillness that is always present within you. It can help to think of this stillness not so much as a stopping of breath but more like an eddy in a flowing stream from which the next breath emerges.

As you lengthen the breath you begin to feel the full rhythmic breathing that flows through your body like a slow-moving, oscillating wave rolling along the spine — loosening your spine from its center and opening the body to its full expression of vitality.

As you inhale, your diaphragm drops down creating more space and expansion in your lungs. As you exhale, your diaphragm rises back up, engaging the muscles of your abdominal core and ribs and clearing the lungs.

It is natural to habitually breathe into your lungs first, expanding and contracting the lungs. With belly breathing, you can focus on drawing a deep breath down into your belly, expanding the belly first and then the lungs. Belly breathing expands the capacity of your lungs.

When you lengthen your exhale, you engage the parasympathetic ('rest and digest') nervous system, lower your heart rate, and increase your sense of relaxation. When you lengthen your inhale, you stimulate the sympathetic ('fight or flight') nervous system which tends to energize the body and increase your heart rate.

Under stress, breath naturally becomes shallow or shortened, depriving the cells of essential oxygen needed for nourishment. By engaging your breath through movement and awareness, deepening your breath, and practicing belly breathing; you can expand the capacity of your lungs, balance the sympathetic/parasympathetic branches of your nervous system, and modulate the stress response allowing the free flow of breath and energy to your cells.

We can use simple breath techniques to help us maintain balance throughout the day. We can calm ourselves and lower cortisol (stress hormone) by focusing on and lengthening the exhale. And when we want to raise our energy, we can focus on the inhale. We can intentionally do this periodically during the day to regulate our levels of stress and balance our energy.

Warming Up the Body Gradually

Every sequence begins with warms-ups that gradually introduce the body to more full movement. The warm-ups gently raise body temperature; soften connective tissue; lubricate the spine and joints with energy, blood, and synovial fluid; and gradually engage the heart and brain. With greater elasticity in the tissues and joints — and energy, breath, and attention engaged — we can safely move into more demanding full-body practices.

Clearing the Energy Channels and Promoting Energy Flow through the Body

Vibrational movements, such as shaking, help us to release held tension and energy blocks within the body and mind; making way for energy to flow and circulate more freely throughout our whole body. Fluid, circular movements help harmonize and balance the energy through the body.

Building Strength and Flexibility in the Musculoskeletal System

When we are young, we may do all kinds of activities that engage the whole of our body like running, jumping, twirling, squatting, etc. As we age, even if we are generally active in our daily life, many of the important muscles that support our stability go unused. The movements and forms in this program are designed to gently strengthen the core and stabilizing muscles upon which balance depends. We awaken and strengthen the whole body, head to toe and into the extremities.

Brain Balancing and Stimulation

Movement arouses and activates our brain. It integrates and anchors new information and experience into our nervous system. It is important that the movements be challenging enough to stimulate the brain and re-awaken connections in the body and consciousness, creating new neural pathways while balancing yin and yang within the body/mind.

There is a saying, "Where the mind goes, energy flows." Many of the movements engage our imagination, drawing our awareness both deeply inward and expansively outward to our surroundings and universe — imagining large effects even when the movements themselves may be subtle. Specific balance poses and movements help us safely practice and challenge our balance with awareness and focus.

Integration and Completion

As you approach completion in your practice, it is important to come back to your center, and acknowledge and integrate your experience, so that what you have learned (mentally, emotionally, and somatically) can move forward into your everyday life.

Upon closing, you can intentionally return to the stillness at the center of your being, connecting with your inherent wisdom; by opening and receiving energy from the universe (nourishing Qi), following a brief moving meditation or guided relaxation, sitting in a moment of silent presence, chanting, or any combination of the above.

"Turn inward, search the body/mind for the unspoiled canvas upon which your life is painted."

Lao-Tsu, Tao Te Ching

VII
The Basic Movements

"Nobody can go back and start a new beginning, but anyone can start today and make a new ending."

Maria Robinson

You will find in this section a background into each of the balance exercises we teach, and some supplemental instruction that may be helpful. However, as it is very difficult to teach movement from a book, our Seniors in Balance practice videos will demonstrate the exercises. These videos may be purchased through our website: seniorsinbalance.com

The movements in the book are shown partially seated and partially standing. However the Seniors in Balance video also demonstrates the standing portion seated in a chair. We always recommend positioning the back a chair in front of you to hold for stability as needed.

In this program we work to:

- Strengthen the stabilizing and core muscles of the body, and fully engage the feet and ankles.
- Establish a sense of grounding and safety
- Create postural awareness
- Engage weight shifting and single leg standing
- Expand range of motion and flexibility
- Integrate breath and movement
- Activate the vestibular system
- Connect eye and body movements
- Widen our visual field of awareness
- Increase sensory awareness
- Move circulation in skin, muscles, and tendons
- Improve counterbalance awareness
- Use cross-lateral, right/left brain hemisphere activity
- Induce the relaxation response
- Nourish energy through organ meridians and primary energy gateways
- Encourage self-acceptance and confidence
- Bring a sense of grounding and safety in the body
- Cultivate presence, openness, receptivity, and enjoyment
- Harmonize the field of energy in your body, mind and spirit

Seated

Preparation

Imagine you are standing at a gate. Take a moment to pause, be present, and set your intention before beginning your practice. Ask yourself: 'What do I want and need from this practice today?', 'what quality of energy will best serve me?'.

Benefits: Pausing before you begin brings your attention to the present, and anchors you in your true reason for practice.

Note: Yoga, Qigong, and Tai Chi practices all begin with a moment to bring oneself present and enter the practice with conscious awareness. In yoga, one may choose a "sankalpa," a clearly stated (often in one word) heartfelt intention. Creating a "sankalpa" is a conscious vow to align ourselves with our highest truth.

Sitting Home (Seated Alignment)

Sit quietly forward and upright in your chair, feel the weight of your body and your pelvis supported by the seat of the chair. Release any tension in your body. Soften your jaw. Let your shoulder blades relax and drop down your back. Connect your awareness to the centerline of your body through your spine. Then bring your awareness to the crown of your head. Imagine a slight lift through your crown. Feel the energy from your crown connecting all the way down through the centerline of your body into your lower abdomen, and grounding all the way through your legs and feet into the earth.

Feel your feet on the floor connecting with the earth. Imagine taproots reaching down into the earth and bringing nourishing earth energy back up though your legs and into your lower abdomen (lower Dantien).

Feel the space within your heart, then all around you (in front, behind, to the sides, above, below). Let your skin soften into this larger space surrounding your body.

Benefits: Induces relaxation and centering in your body. Brings focus, a sense of grounding, and the awareness of energy in your body. Helps establish natural alignment in your spine, allowing greater energy flow through your spine.

Note: Yoga, Qigong, Tai Chi and the harmonious methods of western mind/body movement such as pilates, feldenkeris, Alexander Technique, and Hanna Somatics, all emphasize the importance of being grounded and connected with the earth, establishing your alignment over your center of gravity, moving from your center, and being aware of the flow of energy through the central channel of your body.

Opening to the Natural Breath and Breathing with the Energy Ball

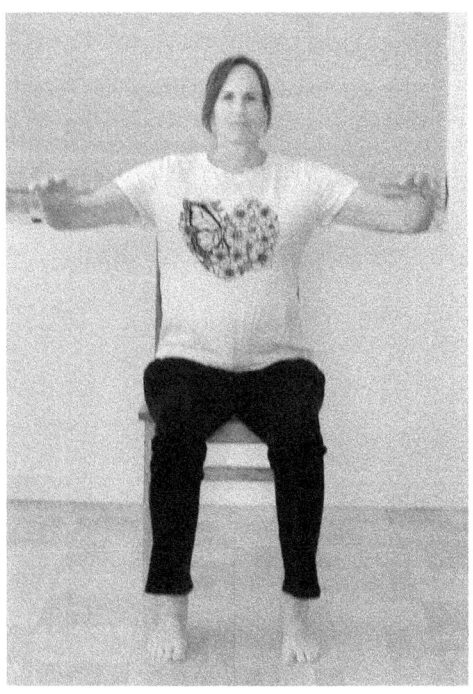

Deepen your inhale and exhale (inhale, expanding your lungs, chest and abdomen; exhale contracting back towards your center). Bring your hands facing each other about six inches apart and held in front of the lower abdomen (lower Dantien or 'Sea of Chi'). Relax your jaw, your shoulders, your elbows. Feel as if there is a ball of energy between your palms, connecting the ball of energy between your palms with the space in your lower abdomen.

Inhaling, let your breath expand, and the space between your hands grow larger, expanding the your abdomen with breath and energy. Exhaling, let your breath flow out of your abdomen, softening back to your center, and compressing the space between your hands. Repeat.

Without force, let your breath roll in and roll out at a slow rhythmic pace. As you breathe, notice the pause at the end of the inhale and at the end of the exhale. Bring your attention to the richness and depth of this pause.

Benefits: Favorable breathing links your body, mind, and emotions; and brings the internal systems of your body into balance. It opens your lungs, oxygenates your cells, activates your parasympathetic (restorative) branch of your nervous system, and restores the acid/alkaline balance of your body chemistry.

Note: Playing with the energy ball and breath in the lower Dantien is common in Qigong. This exercise is also known as 'compressing the Pearl'. The emphasis on the pause at the end of the inhale and exhale helps to naturally lengthen and deepen your breath and create a sense of spaciousness in your mind. It is a practice commonly used in yoga.

Self-massage Patting

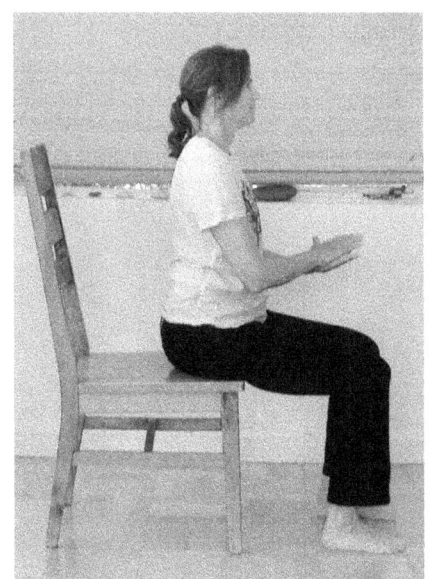
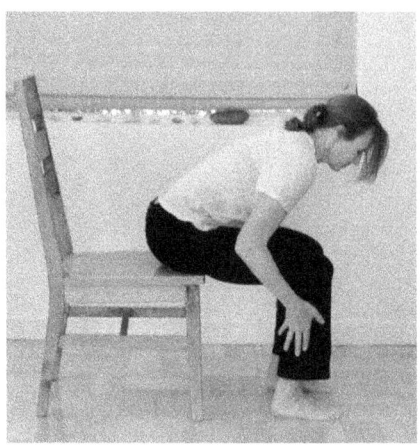
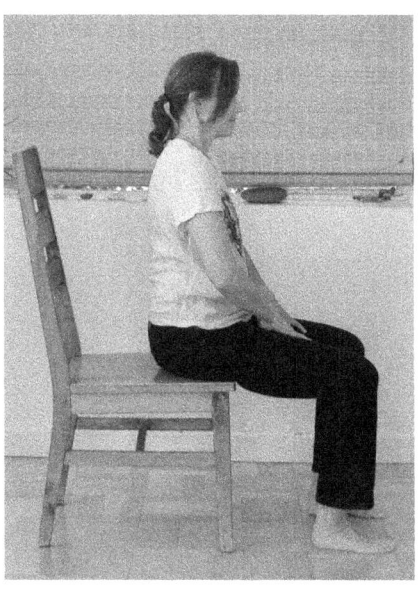
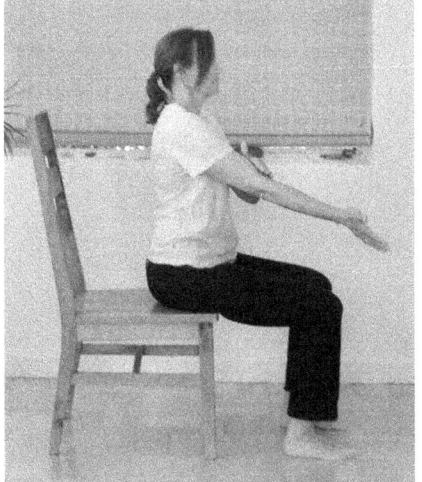

84 | *All About Balance*

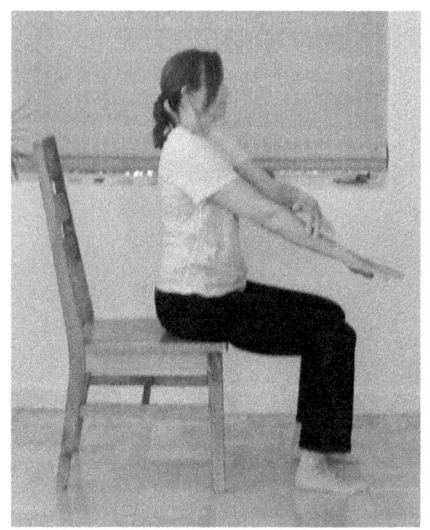
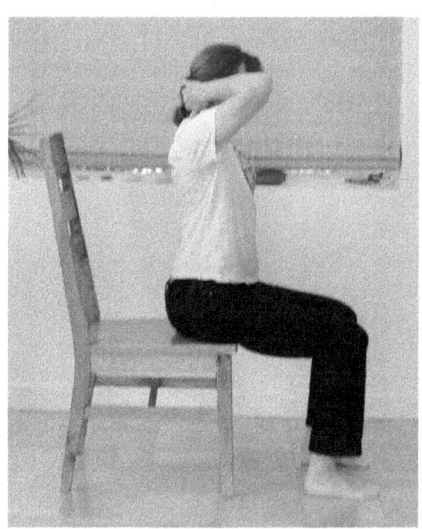
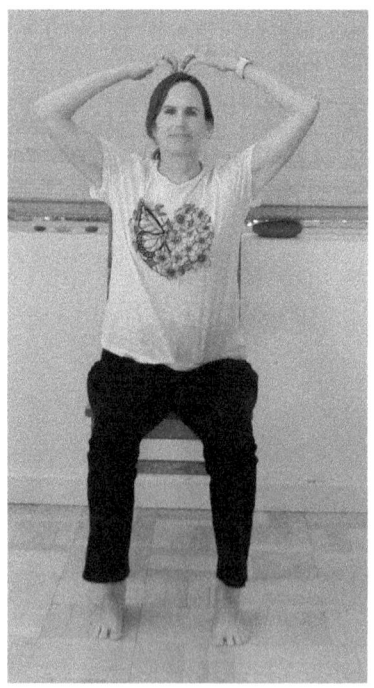

Bring your palms together, rubbing them together in circles to create energy. Gently pat your palms over your kidneys. Then pat down the backs of both legs, around your feet, and up the inside of your legs.

With your fingertips, pat up the centerline of your body to the thymus gland (immune system organ) at the base of the sternum. 'Hum' while gently patting the thymus. Then with the palm of your left hand, pat over to your right shoulder, down the inside of your right arm to your fingertips. Turn your arm over and pat up the backside of your arm, over your shoulder, and across your chest.

Switch arms and pat your left shoulder with your right palm, down the inside of your left arm to your fingertips, up the backside of your arm, and over your shoulder to the center of your chest. With both hands tap the top of your shoulder blades with your fingertips. Then tap up the back of your neck to the base of your scull. Gently tap up to the back of your head. Tap the top of your head at the crown. Gently tap down your face and bring your hands down by your sides.

Benefits: According to Traditional Chinese Medicine (TCM), tapping invigorates your skin and releases energy blockages in your body. Skin stimulation, home to many proprioceptive sensory nerves, enhances overall circulation at this outermost protective barrier of your body.

86 | All About Balance

Note: In Traditional Chinese Medicine body tapping along the energy channels (meridians) and over acupressure points is called Li Da ('tapping with fire'), and is used for moving energy and enhancing overall health. Qigong self-massage can also be done by rubbing your hands along the meridians rather than tapping.

Salute to the Sun (modified for sitting)

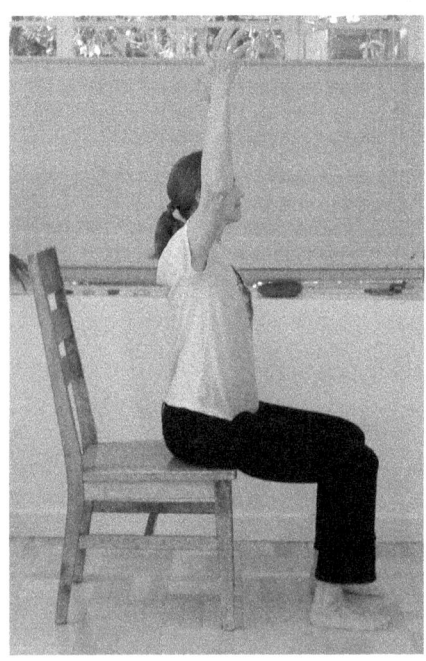
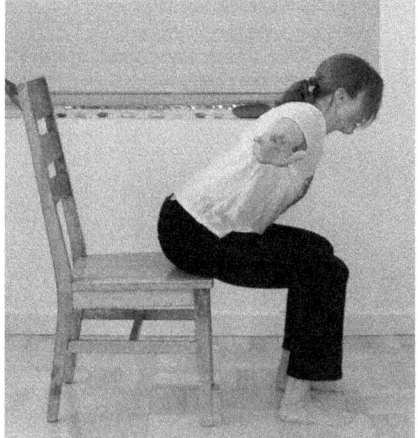
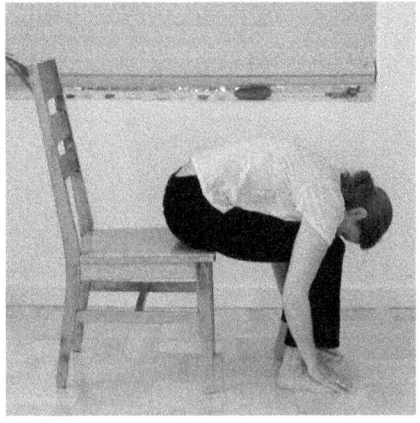

Begin in the Sitting Home position, sitting tall with arms extended down by your sides. Reach your arms out to the sides and up to the sky, looking up to greet the sun, honoring the life-giving energy of the sun. Then with a flat back, fold forward at your hips, resting your upper body on the tops of your thighs.

While resting on your thighs, release your neck and head down. Breathe into the back of your body expanding the space in your spine and releasing any tension there. Then slowly roll up through your spine stacking one vertebrae at a time on top of one another.

Benefit: Brings breath into your whole body, warms up the joints in your vertebral column, awakens movement in your whole spine, creates flow through the channels of energy in your body.

Note: Salute to the sun refers to a basic yoga asana called Surya Namaskara in Sanskrit, meaning 'greeting to the sun'. It is typically done as a standing sequence. Here we are using a modified seated version of the asana. If you cannot rest your body all the way down onto your thighs, that is okay. Use a pillow over your knees, or fold your arms under your chest creating a higher surface upon which to rest. Make sure to release any tension in your head and neck.

Feet and Ankle Stretches and Strengthening

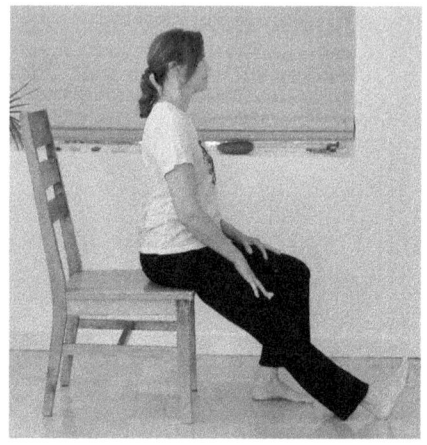

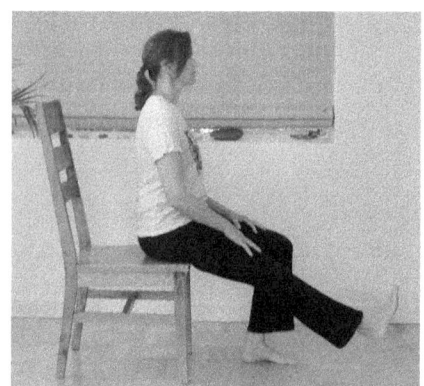

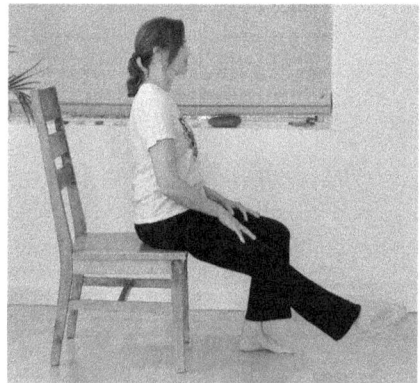

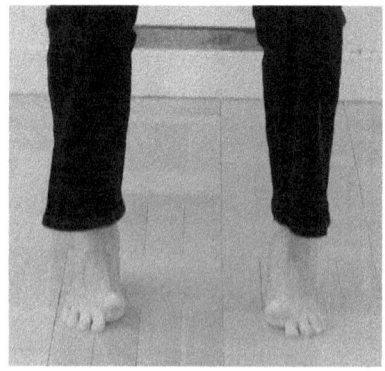

This is most effectively done with bare feet if possible.

Stretch your right leg out long with your heel resting on the floor. Bend your left leg resting your left foot flat on the floor. Sit tall, flex your right foot and tighten your quad muscles at the top of your right thigh (apposing muscle to your hamstrings). Draw your toes toward you, activating the stretch in your foot and ankle. Do not force the stretch. Sit tall to engage a stretch at the back of your leg. Move into it gently with your breath. For those who want a deeper stretch, lean forward gently with a straight spine and hold. If your low back rounds then back off.

When you are done stretching, lift your right leg up straight in front of you about 6" off the floor. Flex and extend your foot. Then draw circles with your foot clockwise, and reverse the direction. Bend your foot side to side strengthening the sides of your ankle. Rest your foot flat on the floor. Lift and lower your big toe while leaving your other four toes on the ground. Then lift and lower your four toes while leaving your big toes on the ground. Rest your right leg on the ground and repeat the sequence on your left side.

Benefits: These movements take your foot and ankle through the full ranges of motion, including big toe plantar flexion which is important for balance. They warm and lubricate your ankle joints and strengthen the muscles of your foot and ankles, bringing aliveness and awareness to your feet.

Note: These movements are influenced by pilates, Feldenkrais, and yoga. Articulating the toes is difficult for many people to do but it helps create conscious connection between your feet and brain, and gets easier with practice. Most people notice feeling steadier, more grounded, and more engaged as they walk after doing a series of exercises focusing on the feet and ankles.

Engaging the Glutes

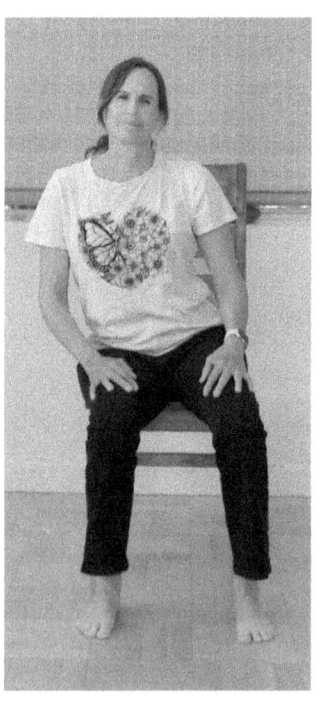
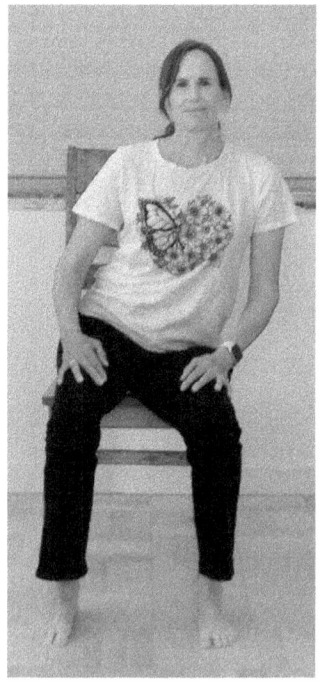

Feel your two sit bones at the base of your pelvis on the chair. Inhaling, press your left foot into the floor, activating the gluteus muscles in your left buttocks and shifting weight onto your right buttocks. Then, exhaling, slowly release your left buttocks back to the chair, and repeat the movement on the other side. Go back and forth shifting side to side (left and right) with the breath.

Benefits: This movement warms up key stabilizing muscles of your body, encouraging strength and flexibility in your lower spine and hips: your obliques (side abdominal muscles), your gluteus medius (hip abductor muscles), your quadratus lumborum (deep lower back muscle), and your erector spinae (lower back muscles). It also gently activates pressure and brings circulation in your feet, ankles, and lower legs. It is a grounding movement, brings our awareness to your pelvic bowl, and activates energy in the lower Dantien.

Seated Spinal Wave

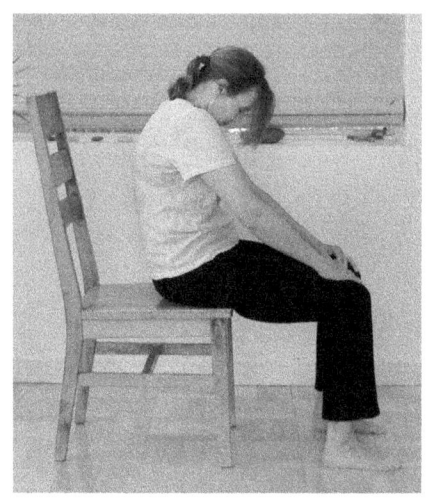
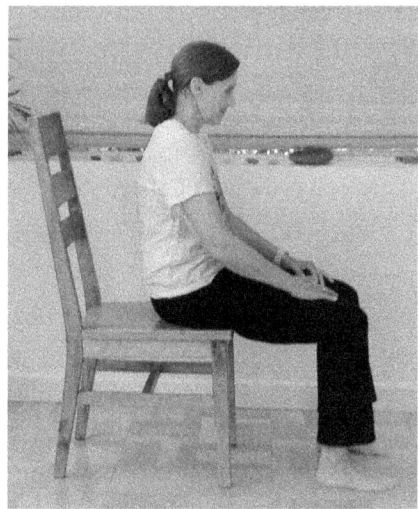
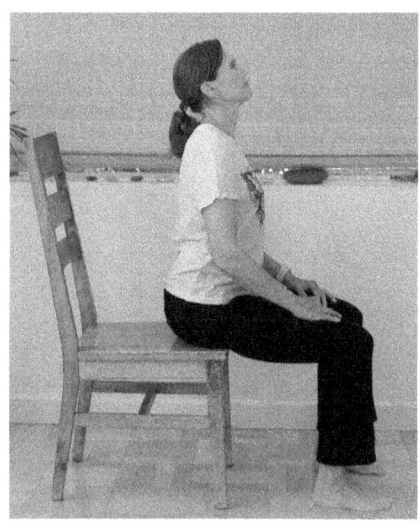
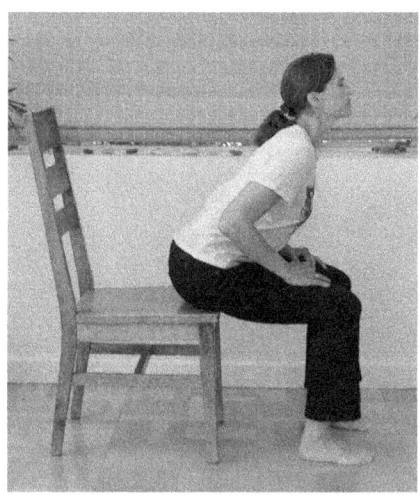

Rest your hands on your thighs. Bring your awareness to the four bony points at the base of your pelvis (left and right sit bones, pubic bone and tailbone). On an exhale, gently rock your tailbone toward your pubic bone, pubic bone toward your belly button, belly button toward your spine; and continue to roll back through your ribcage, upper back, neck, and head tucking your chin to your chest into a comfortable C-curve position; opening the back of the spine.

On the inhale, gently rock your pubic bone towards your chair, and roll through your spine one vertebrae at a time through your abdomen, ribcage, sternum, neck, and head, and gently lifting your chin skyward; opening the front of your spine.

Move fluidly through this movement rolling back and forth like a slow rhythmic ocean wave; inhaling, flowing up onto the shore, then exhaling, and rolling back out and down.

Benefits: According to Qigong, the spinal wave movement opens the gate of life (called the ming men in Qigong) at the center of the waist in the back of the body. Movement at this gate nourishes the kidneys with energy. The spinal wave also encourages an opening of the breath through the torso and warms, loosens, relaxes, and contracts muscles that support the spine bringing blood, nutrients, strength, and flexibility to the spine. The spinal wave activates the supraspinatus muscles along the spine and deep muscles in the pelvic floor and abdominal core, all important for the functional integrity of the spine. This movement balances the ascending (yang) and Descending (yin) energies in the body.

Note: There are different forms of a spinal wave. This movement is similar to the classic cat/cow movement in yoga typically done on all fours to awaken breath and movement in the spine, except it is a continuous flow through the spine.

Gentle Spinal Rotation

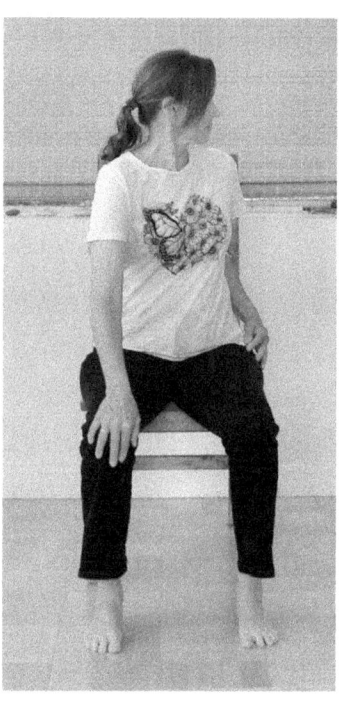 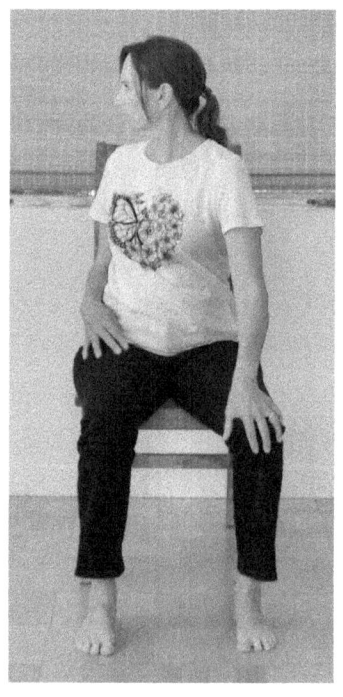

This movement is an extension of the Spinal Wave with a rotation side to side around the central axis of the spine. Exhaling, slide your right hand forward on the thigh toward your knee, and your left hand back toward your body while turning your torso, head, and neck into a gentle twist to the left, looking left. Inhaling, return through the center. Exhaling, slide your left hand forward on your thigh toward your knee, and your right hand back toward your body while turning your torso, head, and neck into a gentle twist to the right, looking right. Repeat the movement back and forth a few times.

Come back to the Sitting Home position, cross your right leg over your left and gently rotate your body to the right. Stop where you feel resistance. Breathe and hold the gentle stretch. You may feel a release as your tissues warm, allowing your body to move into the stretch a little more deeply. Never force the stretch. Repeat this stretch to the other side.

Benefits: This movement takes the spine through rotational movement with the same kinds of benefits as listed for the Seated Spinal Wave.

Note: As you begin the twist, feel the movement originating at the base of your pelvis and rolling up your spine.

Circulating the Pelvis

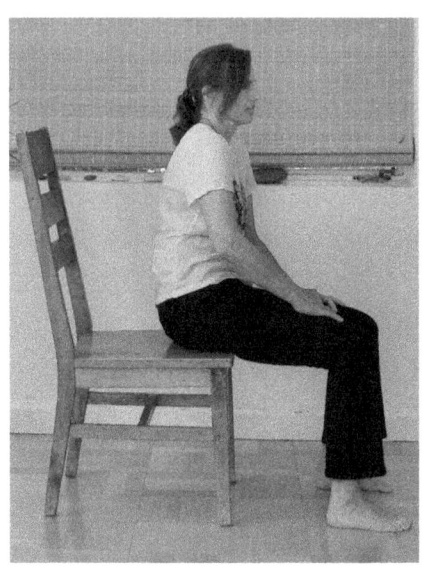 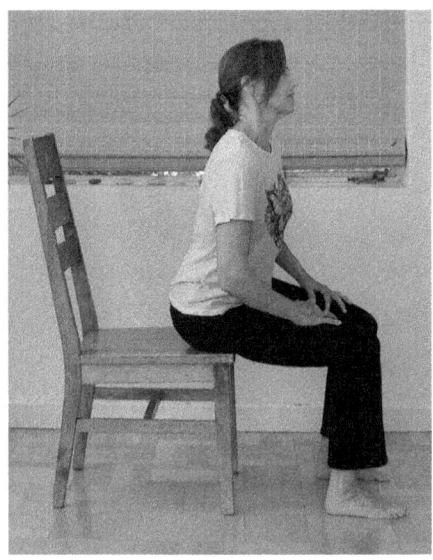

Paying attention to the four bones at the base of your pelvis (see Seated Spinal Wave movement), shift your weight (as in Engaging the Glutes) to your left buttocks (rolling onto the left sit bone). Circle your pelvis around to roll toward your pubic bone. Roll around to your right buttocks (rolling over the right sit bone). Then roll back toward your tailbone. Gently circle your pelvis around a few times in a clockwise direction. Then shift directions and circle the pelvis counterclockwise. Make sure to feel the engagement of your lower abdominal muscles.

Benefits: Strengthens the gluteus muscles in the buttocks and hip, the deep pelvic muscles, the core abdominal muscles, and the oblique muscles used in lateral flexion. These are all key muscles for spinal strength and flexibility, which are key to balance.

Note: This is a very grounding movement (imagine circling the earth) that brings energy into the lower Dantien (typically done standing in Qigong). It is important to engage the deep abdominal muscles as you circle back and release them as you come forward. It is hard for some people to engage the pelvis (tending instead to move from the waist), so emphasis on rolling around the four bones is important.

Circulating the Head

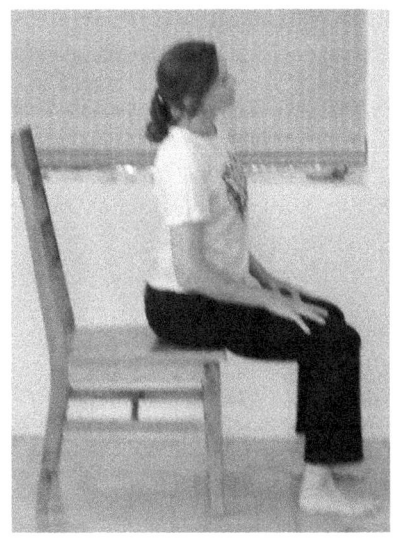 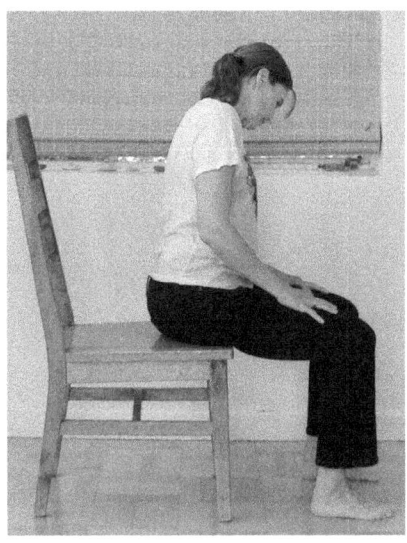

Let your pelvis remain steady in the chair. Begin this movement from your waist and move your head and chest in a clockwise circle. Allow your head, neck, and shoulders to be relaxed and naturally flowing with the movement. Come back to the center and reverse the direction.

Benefits: This movement helps strengthen and create flexibility in the ribcage, thoracic spine, and neck; and strengthens the upper abdominal muscles. It also involves head rotation which engages the vestibular system and proprioceptive sense.

Note: This movement is done subtly and with care to not strain the neck. You can imagine a your head circling the moon, connecting your upper dantien with the larger universe. As you are comfortable, you can move in wider circles. Notice the movement of the thoracic spine and ribcage, being sure to actively engage this area in the movement. Energy is drawn into the upper dantien in this movement.

Chicken Wings with Shoulder Rolls

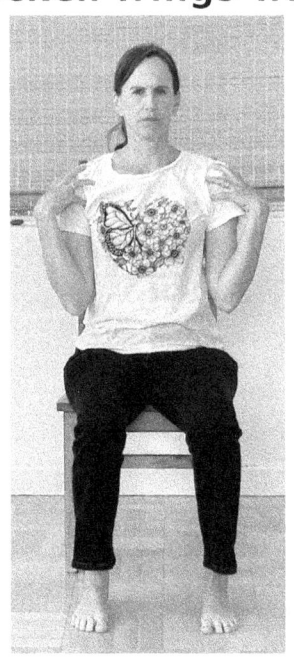
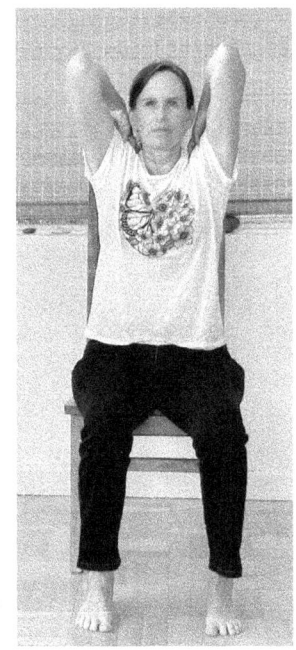

With your hands resting on your shoulders, draw your elbows back, down, and forward in a circular motion, rolling your shoulders. As you draw your shoulders back and down, squeeze your shoulder blades together, using the trapezius muscles between the shoulder blades. Then reverse the direction.

Benefits: The shoulder roll (rotation movement) opens the shoulder joints and ribcage and helps strengthen the latissimus dorsi, trapezius, rhomboid, levator scapula, and pectoral muscles that move the scapula and clavicle. This helps support alignment and release tension in the upper back and neck, and create flexibility in the shoulders. The scapular retractions help teach us how to reach forward and upward while maintaining stability over the body's center of gravity.

Spinal Breathing

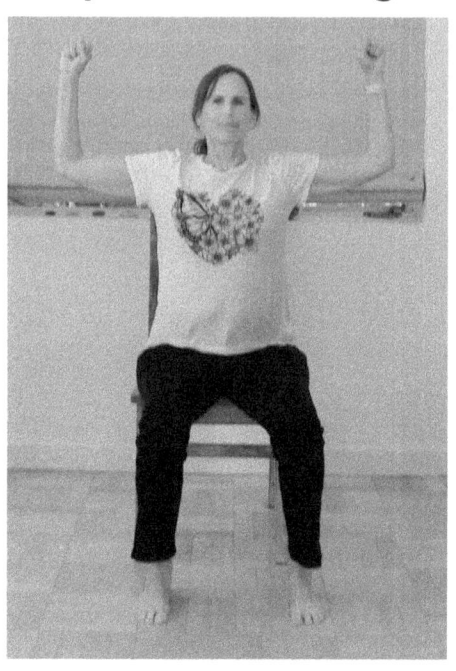

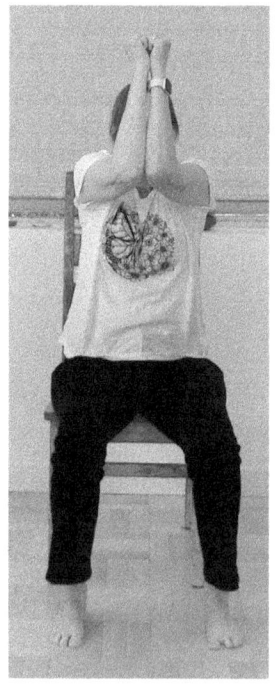
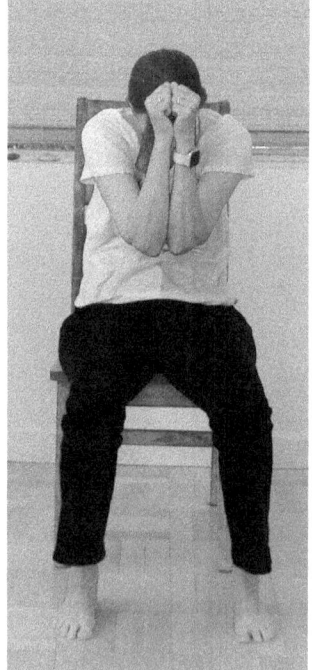

Lift your arms to shoulder height outstretched to the sides of your body. Bend your arms at the elbow upwards 90 degrees as if creating a goalpost. On an exhale, draw the lower parts of your arms together in front of your body to touch while keeping your arms raised. Then tuck your elbows down towards your abdomen, engaging your abdominal core muscles. As you inhale, draw your elbows back up and out to the sides opening the chest, front of the spine, and neck. Move back and forth opening up and out on the inhale and tucking in and down on the exhale.

Benefits: This movement has multiple benefits in that it strengthens the core muscles in the abdomen (the rectus abdominus), opens the shoulder joints and ribcage, and helps strengthen the latissimus dorsi, trapezius, rhomboid, levator scapula, and pectoral muscles that move the scapula and clavicle. This helps support alignment and core strength, and release tension in the upper back and neck.

Crossovers

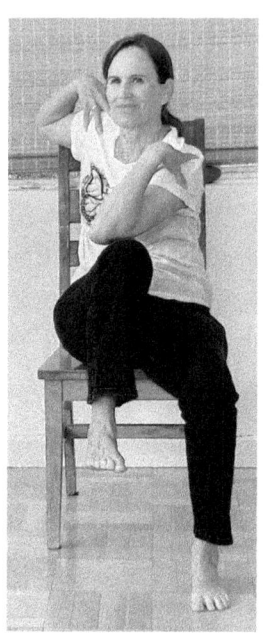

Rest your hands on your shoulders. Draw your left elbow across your body and down to your right thigh. Meanwhile lift your right leg up to meet the elbow. Then return your leg and elbows back to center. Draw your right elbow across your body to meet your left thigh. Repeat back and forth a few times.

Benefits: While sharing similar benefits to the Chicken Wing movements above, this exercise is also a cross-lateral movement activating both sides of the brain. It is a full body movement — involving bending, rotation of the spine, and arm and leg movements, all while turning the head and being supported by the chair. It stregthens the abdominal core and quad muscles in the thighs. It also activates the vestibular system and the proprioceptive sense, and encourages left and right hemisphere integration.

Arm Stretches

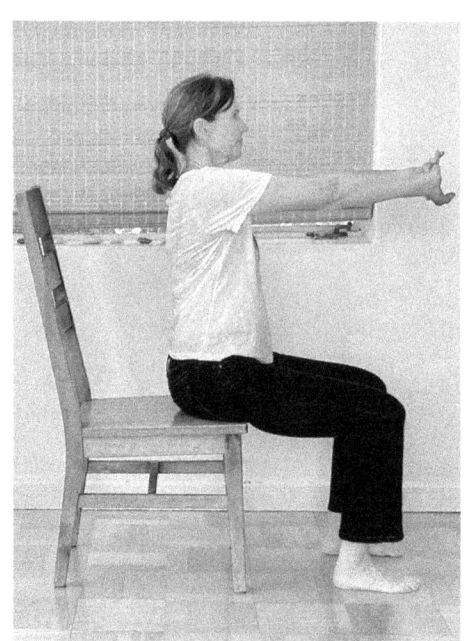
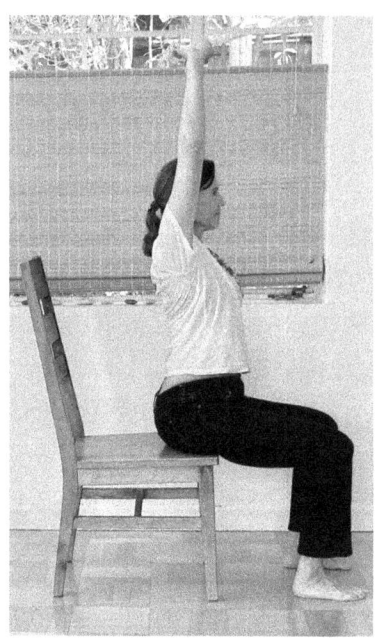
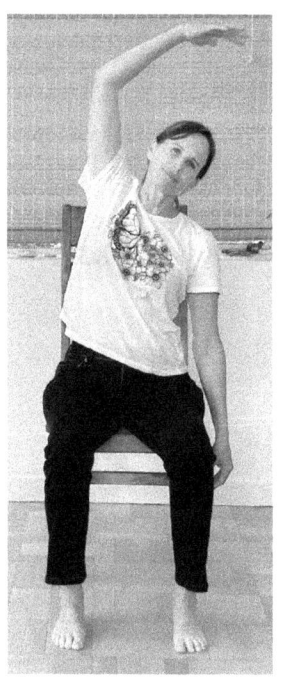
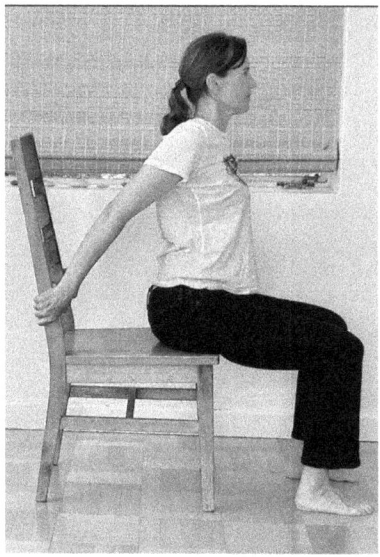

Intertwine the fingers of both hands. Roll them over to face outward from your body. Stretch your arms out in front of you from the wrist, the elbows, and the space between the shoulder blades.

Then draw your hands up overhead, pressing your palms against the sky and stretching upward. Let your right hand float down to your side. Reach up slightly with your left hand (to create length in the left ribs) and gently stretch over to the right side. Open the side of your ribs and breathe into the stretch. Then let the left hand float down to your side. Take a moment to breath and center. Then repeat the movement to the other side.

Reach behind you with both hands and grasp the sides of the chair. Gently squeeze the shoulder blades together and open the chest.

Benefits: These movements release tension in the arms, shoulders, and wrists and open the chest and upper back. Many of us, after years of sitting, have a somewhat restricted chest and curved upper back. This movement helps bring flexibility to this area.

Wide Leg Stance with Shoulder Stretches

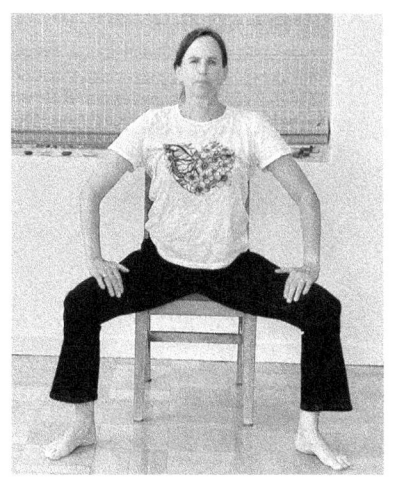 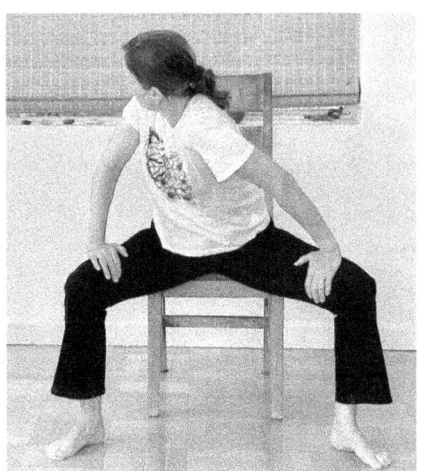

Open your legs out wide, with your knees bent and feet resting flat on the floor. Place your hands on your thighs just before the knees. Press your left hand against your left thigh while rolling your left shoulder forward and straightening the arm as much as possible. Rotate your body to the right, looking over your right shoulder.

Breathe into the stretch. Then return back to center. Repeat the movement on the other side, rolling the right shoulder forward and rotating left. Return back to center.

Benefits: This movement stretches the groin muscles; activates the gluteus and leg muscles; takes the spine into rotation; shifts the body side to side while turning the head in space; and engages the vestibular system and proprioceptive sense. It also helps move lymph concentrated in the groin.

Elephant Sprays Water

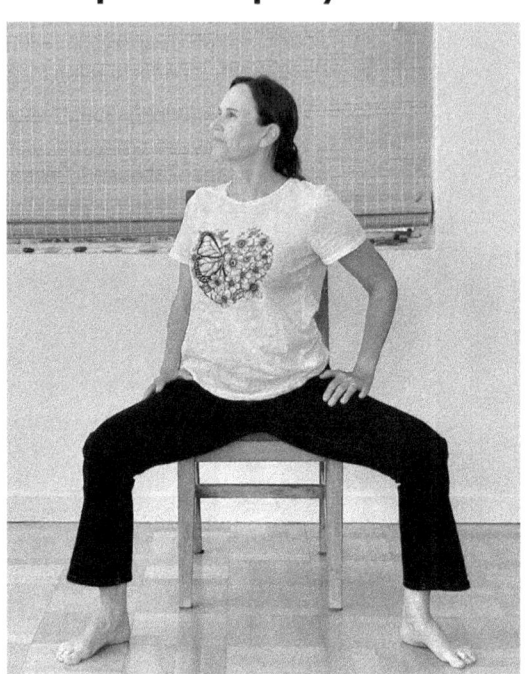

Still in the wide leg stance with knees bent, place your hands to rest just above and on the inside of your thighs. Imagine you are an elephant with a large trunk. Turn your torso to your right, lifting through the sternum at the center of the chest, looking right. Raise your head as if raising your trunk overhead.

Leading with your sternum, swoop your body down and across to your left leg. Look up and lift through the sternum. Repeat the movement back and forth side to side.

Benefits: This Elephant movement activates the vestibular system in the inner ear. It is a whole-body,

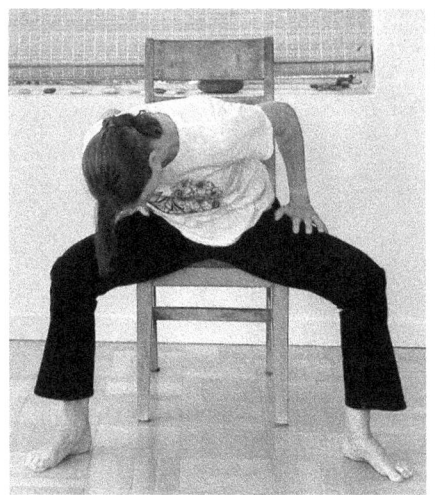
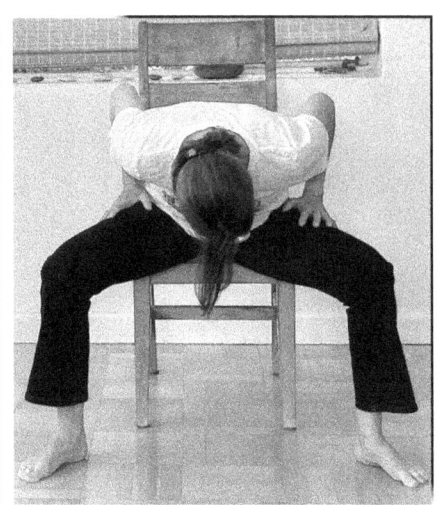
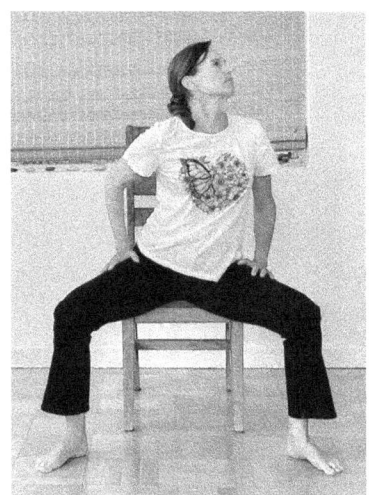

side-to-side movement which encourages flexibility in the spine.

Note: This movement is a seated adaptation of a Qigong movement from the 8 Brocades Qigong form.

Sit to Stand

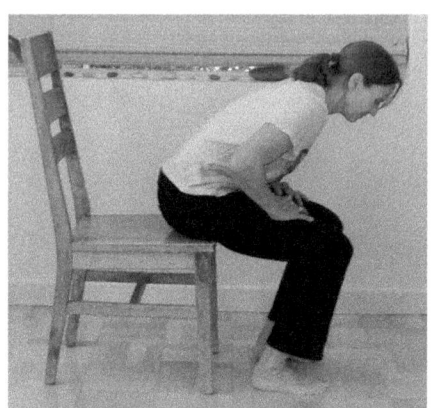
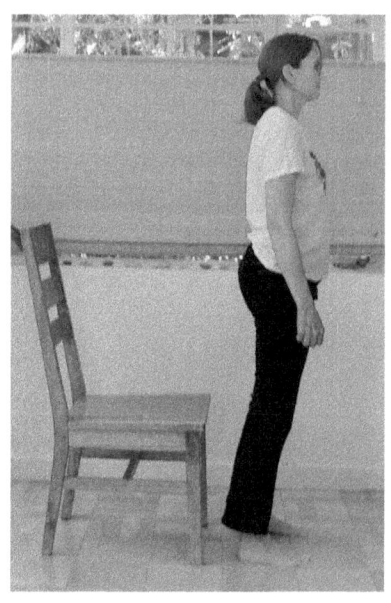
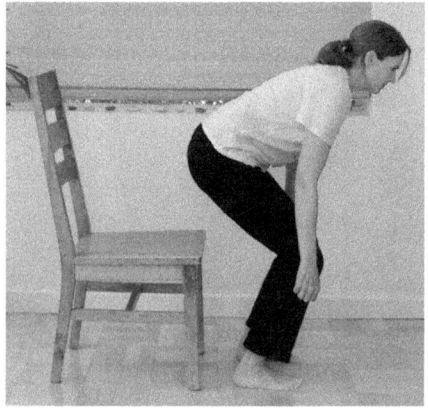

Move your heels back towards your chair to a bit behind your knees. Squeeze the muscles in your buttocks (gluteus muscles) to engage the stabilizing muscles in the legs. Lean forward, shifting your weight over your center of gravity, and engage the deep muscles in your lower abdomen. Looking towards the floor, slowly bring yourself to standing, rolling up the spine, stacking one vertebrae on top of another

Benefits: This movement is an exercise in activating and strengthening the stabilizing muscles of the body to effectively and consciously raise the body from sitting to standing, and establishing stability over the base of support.

Note: The Sit to Stand movement is an essential component of balance as it is a significant fall risk for seniors. It can be practiced repeatedly to build strength and awareness. For some seniors, it may be easier to stand when widening the legs, using more of the muscles in the back of legs.

Standing

Standing Mountain Pose (Tadasana)

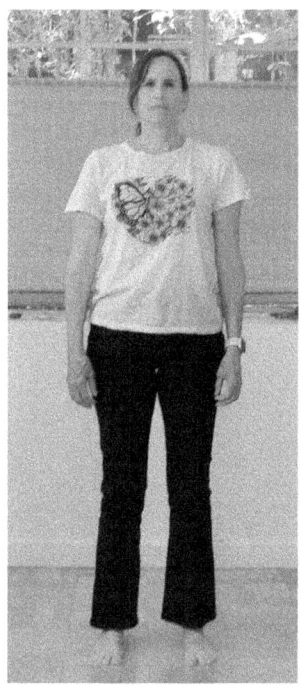

Stand with your feet hip-width apart. Feel roots extend from your lower abdomen down into the earth, rooting into the earth. Let your knees be easy (not locked), and shoulders soft. Imagine a cord gently lifting the top of your head (crown) upward aligning the vertebrae of your spine like a string of pearls. Let your chin release back over your shoulder girdle to relieve tension in the neck. Let your pelvic bowl soften down to release any tension in the lumbar spine. .

Benefits: The Mountain Pose opens the central energy flow through the spine from the tailbone through the crown of the head. The aim is to have a relaxed but engaged stance (effortless action).

Note: Standing in Mountain Pose (Tadasana) is an important asana in yoga. Qigong also has a version of standing called Wu ji. Everyone's spinal posture is different. The intent is to stand with greater ease, and build rather than deplete energy while standing. The lift at the crown of the head is not a forced lifting but a gentle prompt to feel a sense of spaciousness and softness through the spine between the tailbone and crown.

Qigong Shaking

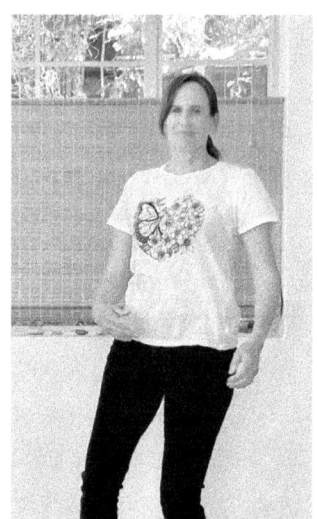

Widen your feet a little more than hip width apart. Relax your arms and let them hang like loose ropes to the sides of your body.

Gently begin to shake up and down, releasing any tension you may feel head to toe. You can shake out your voice clearing energy and activating the vagus nerve, by sounding ('ahhh,' 'mmm,' whatever feels good) and feel the sound vibrate through your body. Then come back to stillness.

Benefits: Qigong Shaking loosens held tension in the body, muscles, and joints; promotes an exchange of Qi throughout the body; increases circulation; helps regulate the nervous system; and engages a childlike sense of playfulness and freedom. The sound vibration helps tone the Vagus Nerve.

Note: The shaking exercise is a common practice in Qigong. It activates the flow of energy through the connective tissue (fascia) in the body. It is also an energy balancing practice.

Twist and Pat

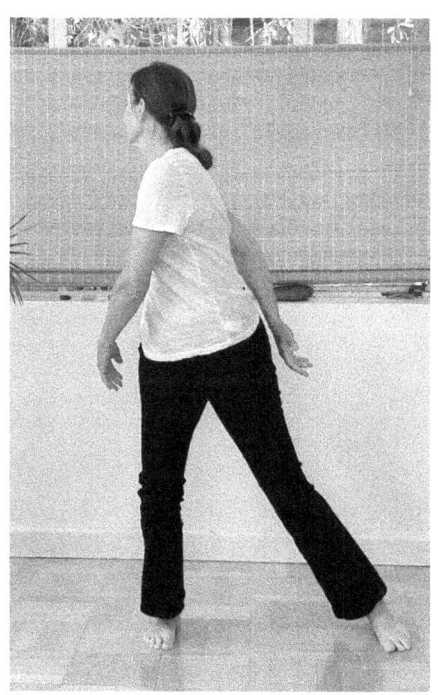
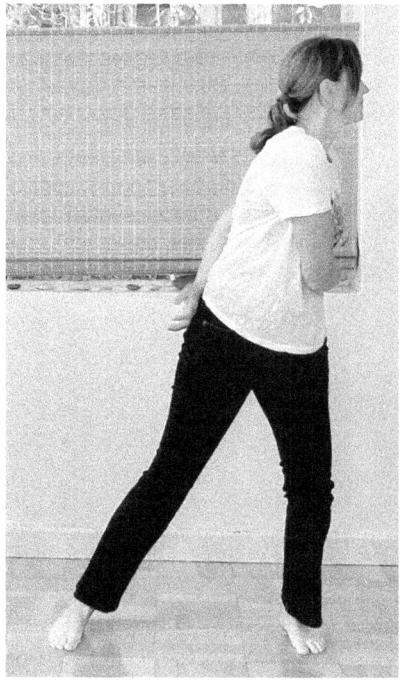

Widen your stance. Shift your weight to your right leg, then to your left leg, bending the weighted knee while turning your torso. Let your arms begin to swing, like loose ropes gaining momentum, out naturally from your body, following the turning of your torso. As your arms swing around, let your hands tap your body (the back hand to the kidney). Move side to side, shifting your weight and swinging your torso and arms around your body as you move.

Benefits: Twist and Pat is a weight-shifting exercise using the strength of the legs. It stimulaties the kidney and liver meridians. It moves the head side to side through space, activating the vestibular system; and circulates energy through the legs and into the lower Dantien. It's is a rotational movement through the spine increasing flexibility and releasing tension in the upper body.

Note: Twist and Pat is a common Qigong/Tai Chi practice, often done to warm up the body, balance the nervous system, clear energy, and loosen the joints.

Dropping the Post (Heel Lift and Drops)

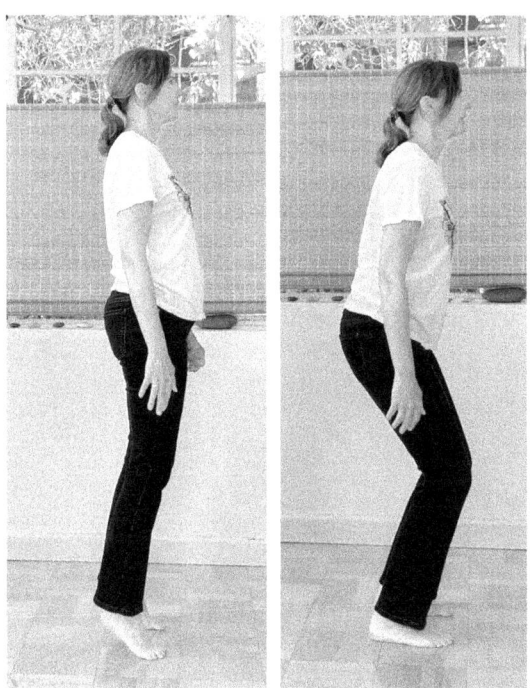

Begin in the Mountain Pose. Come up on your toes and drop your heels to the ground with some force creating a vibration through your body. Repeat lifting up and dropping down.

Benefits: The impact of the heel drop stimulates the bones in the lower body (particularly the hip). It strengthens the calf muscles in the ankles, creates flexion in the foot and toes, and is a moving balance practice.

Note: Anyone who is not confident in their balance should hold onto the back of a chair for support while doing this movement.

Modified Squats with Arms

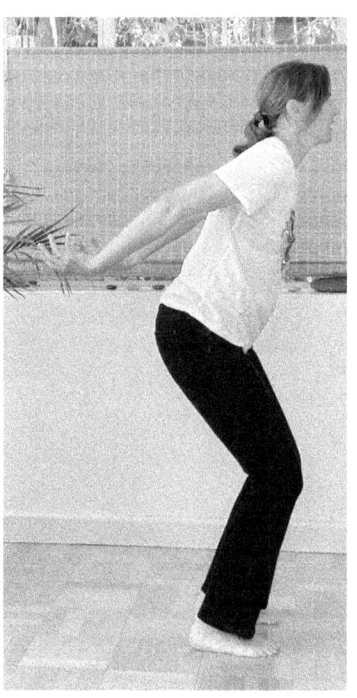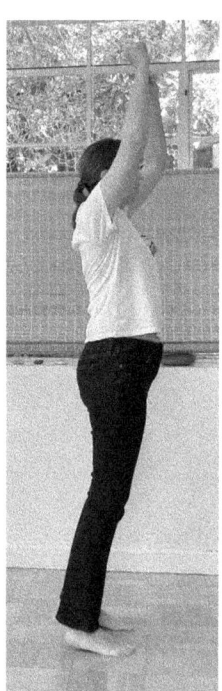

Stand with your feet hip-width apart and your arms by your sides. Drop into your knees, letting your weight shift into your heels, while swinging your arms backwards. Then come up onto your toes while swinging your arms forward and out front to shoulder height. Swing back and forth.

Benefits: Modified squats strengthen the stabilizing leg and core muscles of the body. They deepen and expand the breath, raising the heart rate slightly and circulating energy flow in the body.

Note: This is a challenging moving balance exercise. For anyone with balance challenges, simply hold the back of a chair while swinging one arm. You can also leave your feet on the ground while gently shifting your weight back to front for greater stability. For anyone with high blood pressure move slowly as this exercise can raise your heart rate.

Five-Pointed Star

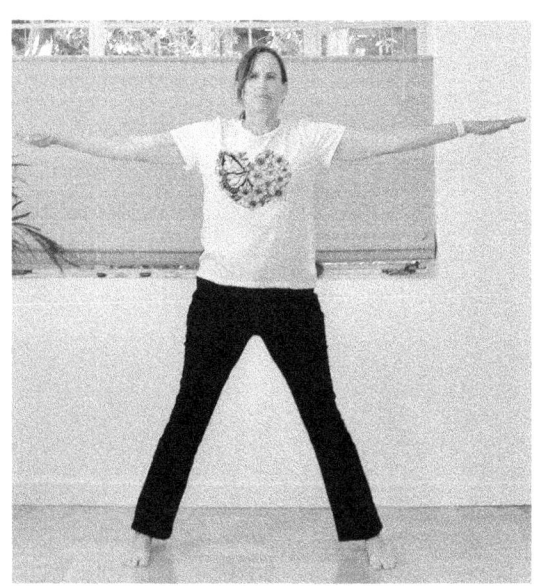

Step out from the Mountain Pose into a wide leg stance, straighten your legs to a soft knee position (straight but not locked). Extend your arms out to the sides as if touching the horizon. Feel the strength of this pose. Feel the sense of energy radiating from your heart out your arms, down your legs, and up through the crown of your head; and receiving energy from the universe in all directions back to your heart center.

Benefits: The five-pointed star evokes a sense of whole body grounding and expansion, as well as postural stability and alignment. It strengthens the legs; opens the heart, chest, and lungs; and promotes energy flow through the whole body.

Note: This is a traditional standing pose in yoga (called 'Utthita Tadasana' in Sanskrit) often done as a transition into the warrior poses.

Goddess

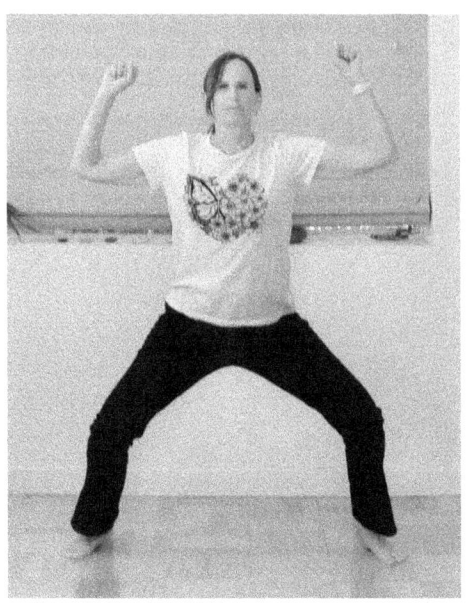

From the Five-Pointed Star, turn both heels inward while simultaneously bending the knees, and bending the elbows 90-degrees upward. As you come down into the pose make the sound, 'haaa.' Return upright and repeat.

Benefits: This is a strengthening and stabilizing movement for the legs and buttocks (gluteus muscles). It opens the hips, shoulders, and chest. The 'ha' sound is a sound related to the heart, and in Qigong is said to calm the heart and release emotional tension.

Note: The goddess is a yoga pose that evokes feminine energy often seen in ancient statues. The seniors we teach like making a powerful vocal sound of 'ha' as a group. It is playful and revitalizing.

Warrior 1 (Lunge)

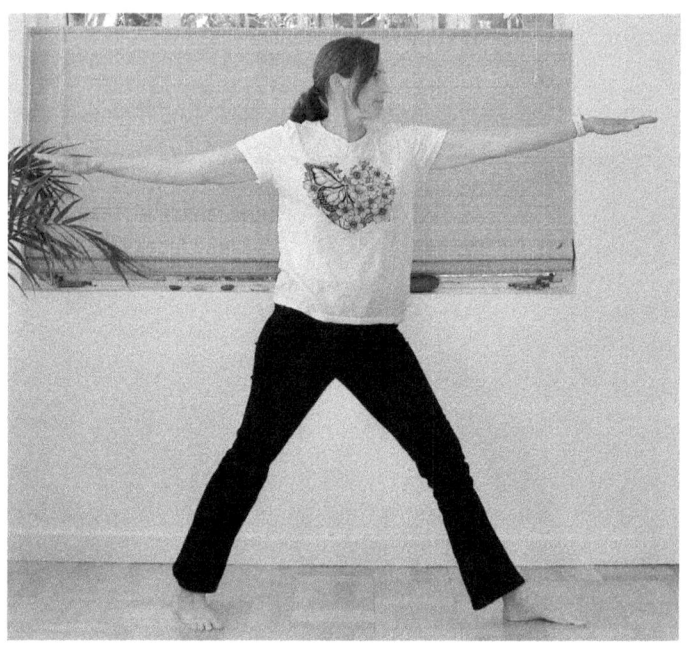

From the Mountain Pose, turn to your right, and step forward a few feet with your left leg so both legs are straight. Your left foot is pointing left and your back right foot is angled 45 degrees outward. Bend your left knee, leaving the back right leg straight. Make sure your left knee is over your ankle (not forward of it) to protect the knee joint. Raise your arms up overhead in a somewhat rounded soft position, keeping your shoulders relaxed. Feel the lengthening of your spine, and the stretch at the back of your left leg. The more you ground into the earth through your legs, the more lift you will feel rising upwards. Hold the pose for a breath or two, and then let your arms float back to your sides. Repeat the movement to the other side.

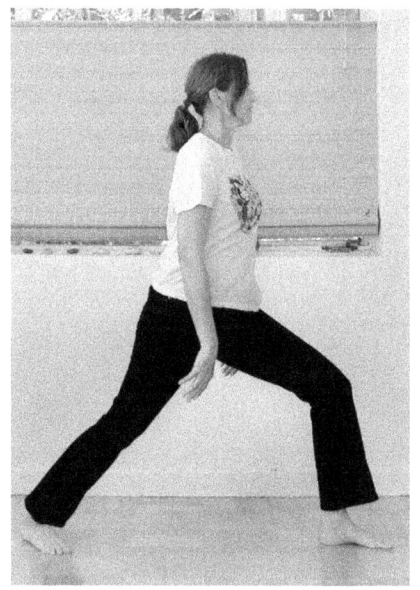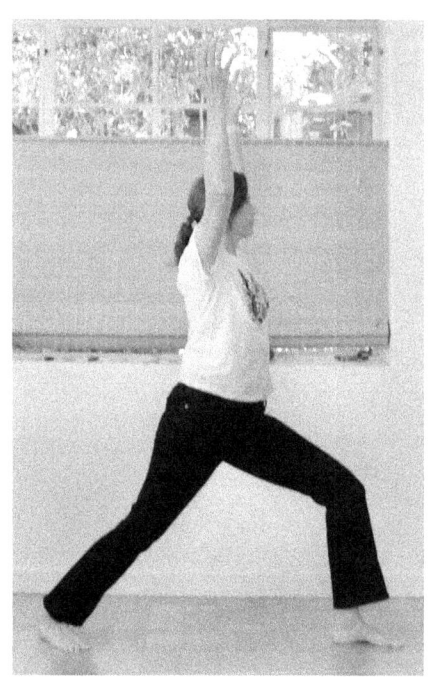

Benefits: The warrior poses are about cultivating strength, confidence and focus. Warrior 1 creates strength and flexibility in the lower legs and pelvis, and in the spine. It also creates expansion upward (rising out of the grounded strength of the lower body) and an opening in your center (solar plexus chakra)

Note: If unsure of your balance, you can stand behind a chair and use the chair to stabilize and extend one arm up at a time. Warrior 1 ('Virabhadrasana') is part of the classic warrior series of yoga poses.

Scoop the Sea, Look at the Sky

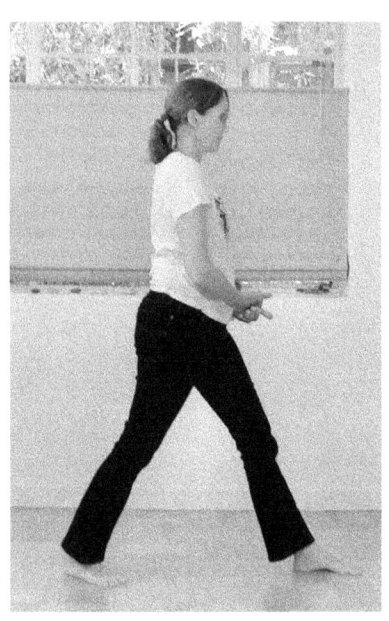
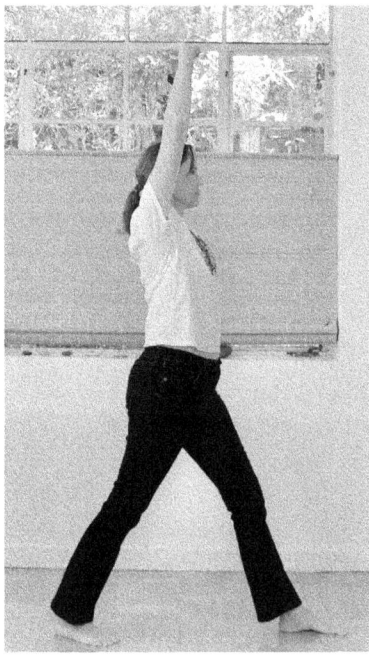
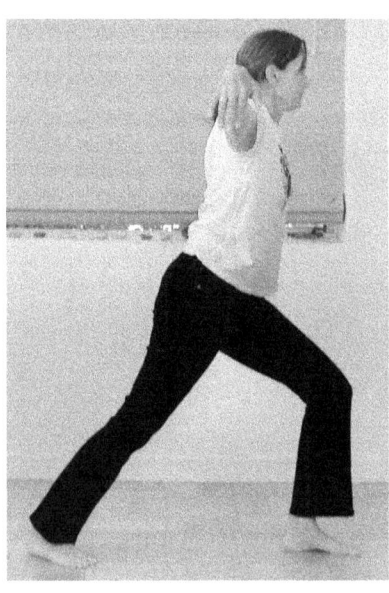
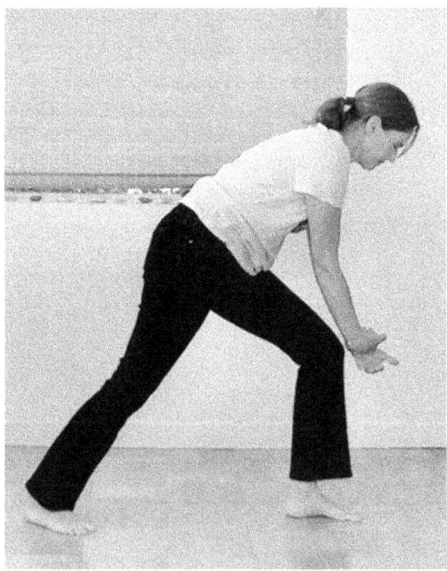

From the Mountain Pose, turn to your left and step forward a few feet with your left leg so both legs are straight. Your left foot is pointing forward and your back right foot is pointed about 45 degrees outward (similar to warrior 1). Place your hands one palm atop the other (though not touching) in front of your lower abdomen. Inhaling, draw your hands up the front centerline of your body, rolling your palms over at the heart, and bringing your hands palm face up (still stacked) overhead. Let your hands separate and come down by your sides to shoulder level. Exhale, drop your wrists, and let your arms continue downwards while bending your left knee. Bring both arms around and down to scoop the sea, palms stacked one over the other. Then inhaling, draw your hands up through the centerline of your body to overhead as you straighten your right leg. Repeat the movement flowing with the breath.

Benefits: This is a wonderful whole body movement with benefits for balance. It opens and strengthens the front and back of the spine. It strengthens the legs coming forward into the lunge. And creates extension and strength through the arms. It balances yin, and yang energies, and activates the vestibular and proprioceptive senses.

Note: For greater stability, you can hold the back of a chair .

Horse Stance

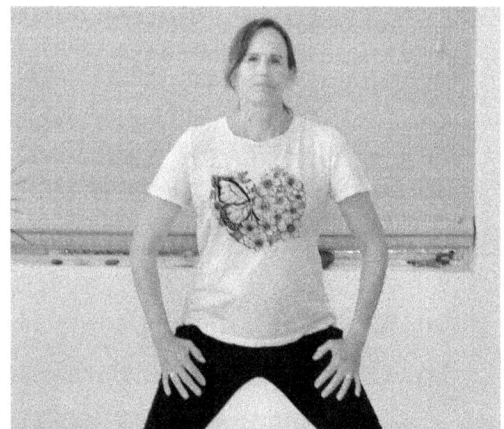

Come into the Mountain Pose. Inhale and open your stance to a bit wider than hip-width apart. Bend your knees. Feel as if you are going to sit in a chair. Your tailbone is extending back toward the wall behind, with your upper body upright.

Benefits: The horse stance is very strengthening for the legs and torso, and brings energy into the lower Dantien.

Note: The horse stance is a very common stance from which many Tai Chi moves begin; it can be a physically challenging exercise in itself to hold the horse stance position for a while. How challenging it is depends on how low you bend your knees and how long you hold the posture. What is appropriate will be different for every person. Holding the back of a chair often makes it easier and more stable for seniors to lower their stance, engaging and strenghtneing the muscles of the legs.

Pulling the Bow

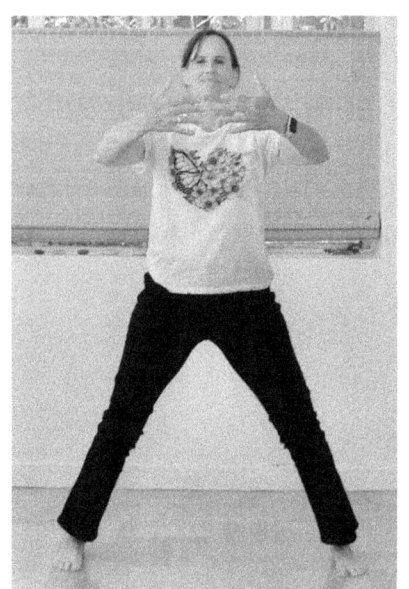
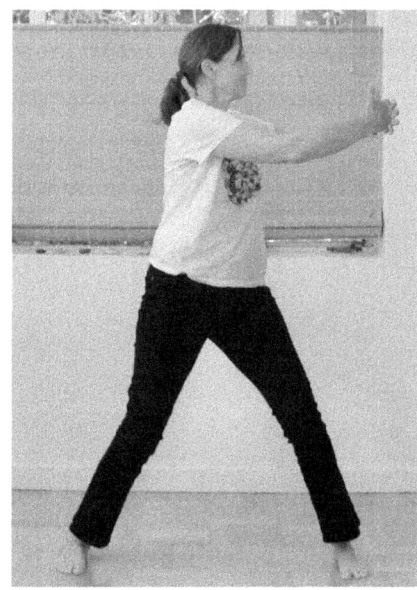
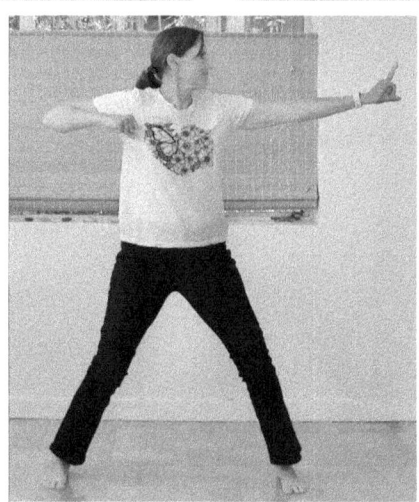

From Horse Stance, bring your arms around in a circle as if embracing a tree. Turn your torso left, holding the tree. Extend your left arm to the left, and point your left index finger upwards to the sky. At the same time, make a fist with your right hand and pull your fist across your right cheek. Let your eyes follow the tip of the pointed right index finger. Pause in this position. Bring your arms back to embrace the tree and turn back towards the center. Repeat the movement to the other side. Then step back into the Mountain Pose.

Benefits: This movement has many benefits. Pointing the index finger stretches and opens the large intestine meridian that runs from the index finger up the forearm. It's helpful for detoxifying the digestive organs, balancing the fluids of the body, and releasing tension and blocked emotions.

The Horse Stance strengthens the stabilizing and core muscles of the body. Pulling the bow stretches and strengthens the arms.

Note: Pulling the Bow comes from one of the oldest Qigong sequences called the 'Eight Silk Brocades' or 'Ba Duan Jin'. It was practiced by the Shaolin monks for physical strength and mental focus.

Walking the Line

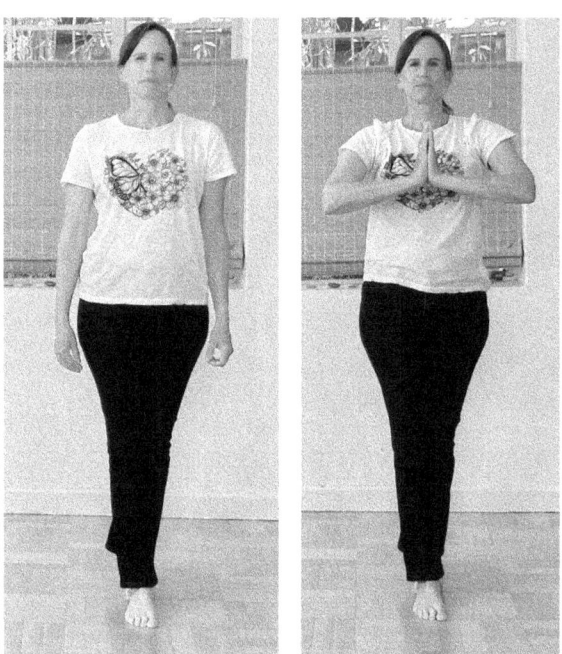

Begin in the Mountain Pose. Shift your weight to the left. Step your right foot to the right and forward of your left foot so your right heel is in the same line as the tip of your left toes. Slowly walk (heel to toe) your right heel to be lined up directly in front of your left foot (both pointing forward). Bring your weight to rest equally between both legs.

If balanced confortably raise your arms overhead. Take a few breaths here and then bring your palms together and draw your hands down your centerline in front of your heart (Anjali Mudra/prayer hands). Use a chair for support if uncertain of your balance.

Benefits: This is an excellent practice for balance. It strengthens the intricate muscles in the feet, ankles, and lower legs — creating stability in our foundation. By narrowing the base of support, we challenge our proprioceptive senses and exercise the capacity to continually rebalance ourselves (postural re-weighting).

Note: this is a classic balancing move. If your balance allows you take this pose further, you can practice taking a few steps forward rolling heel to toe, and backwards toe to heel as if walking a single line.

Modified Tree

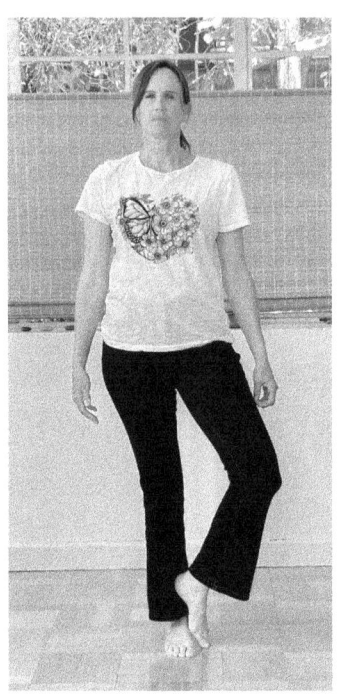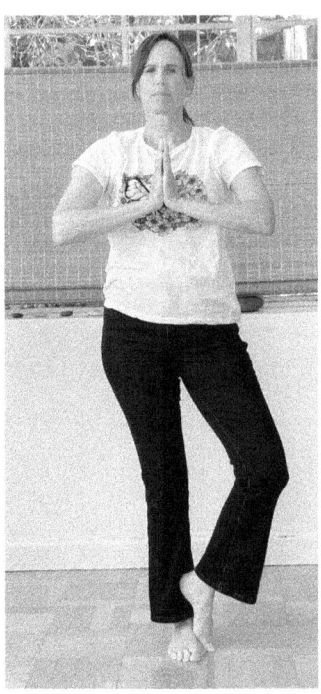

Begin in the Mountain Pose. Connect with the line of energy running from above the crown of your head, through the centerline of your body, and down into the earth. Imagine there are roots running down from your lower abdomen, through the legs and, into the earth like a tree.

Shift your weight fully onto your right leg. Slide the big toe of your left foot over to your right ankle and, with your big toe anchored on the ground, rest the heel of your left foot over your ankle. Rest on a fixed point before you. Let your pelvis be stable (neither in flexion or tucked). Your shoulder blades are relaxed down your back.

Once you feel steady in your balance, let your arms come up with an inhaling breath, extended out to the sides, then up overhead. Pause to hold the pose, breathing. Then draw your hands, palms together, overhead and exhaling, bring them down the centerline of your body to your heart.

Benefits: The Tree Pose brings strength in the legs, feet, and pelvis, as well as the mind. It helps improve our capacity for standing on one leg, and remaining rooted and steady on the earth, while opening the upper body and focusing the mind. The movement of the arms opens the upper back between the shoulder blades. The hand gesture at the end stretches the wrists; directs energy to the heart, chest, and lungs; and balances the right and left hemispheres of the brain. After practicing this in a class of seniors, there is often a palatable calm, focused energy in the room.

Note: The tree pose is a classic balancing asana in yoga called 'Vrikshasana.' The hand gesture (mudra) with hands together in front of the heart is called the Anjali mudra. There is a focus on harmonizing energy and awareness through the central line of the body.

Hold the back of a chair for stability as needed.

Golden Cock Stands on One Leg

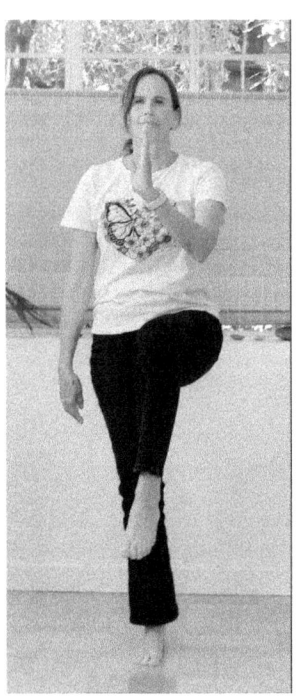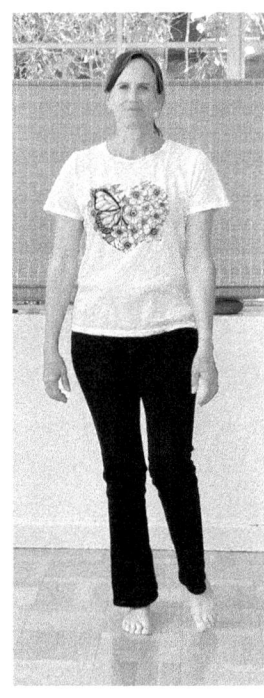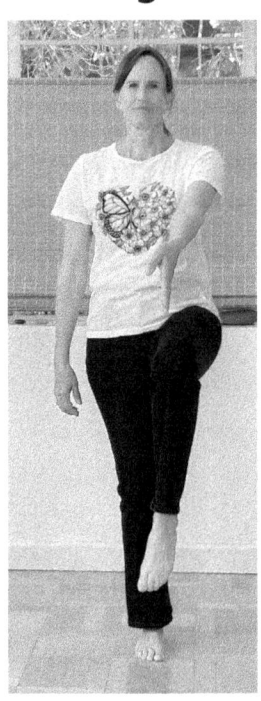

Begin with your feet hip-width apart. Shift all of your weight to your right leg, and bend your left knee up in front of you to a 90 degree angle. Let your left toes hang downward. Then begin shifting your weight back to the left letting your left toes land on the ground first, sinking your weight into your left leg while bending the right leg to 90 degrees.

Repeat the weight shifting and lifting of the leg back and forth. Once you feel balanced enough in this movement, add your arms as follows: Bring your left hand in front and perpendicular to your left knee, with your hand cocked downward. As you lift your left knee to the bent position, lift your left hand just above your knee as if lifting the strings of a puppet. Your hand rises with the knee, and gradually tilts to a cocked upward position.

Let your eyes be soft. This is a very challenging moving practice to work up to. We recommend using the back of a chair for stability, making sure to find your balance using the legs before adding the arm movements. It can also be helpful to practice weight shifting before lifting the legs.

Benefits: This movement is excellent for directly challenging balance while moving. It activates the vestibular system and proprioceptive senses. It strengthens the leg muscles and creates mind focus.

Note: This is a classic Qigong practice known as 'Jin Ji Du Li.' Qigong masters claim it is a powerful practice that creates complete circulation of blood and Qi through the body, rebalancing the internal organs. Done correctly, energy moves through the six meridians in the legs, concentrating in the bubbling spring point at the bottom of the feet. Being a challenging balance practice, we recommend seniors have a chair nearby and use it as necessary.

Pressing Earth and Sky

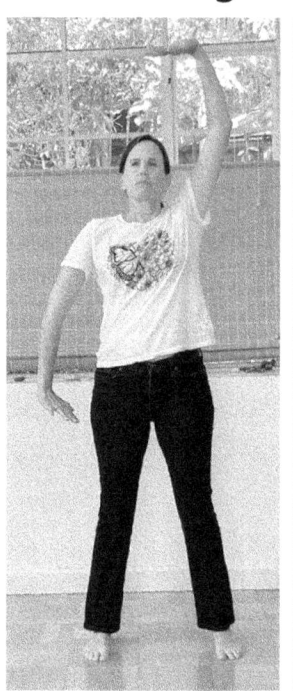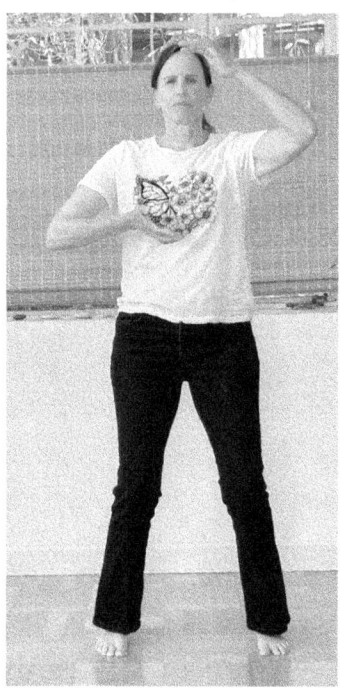

From the Mountain Pose, bring your hands facing each other as if holding a ball in front of your heart. Turn your right hand, palm facing down to the earth, and press the right palm down by your thigh with your fingers pointing toward the thigh (pressing the earth). At the same time, draw your left hand, palm facing upward, up your body. Roll your palm all the way over to extend up to the sky, palm pressing the sky. Press the earth and press the sky.

Then turn your palms toward each other and draw them closer to each other, passing in front of the heart and continuing the movement to the other side.

Benefits: This movement stretches the upper spine, and regulates energy flow in the spleen (which governs blood flow in the body). Bringing the sky energy down and the earth energy up merges yin and yang energies in the heart.

Note: This movement is part of the classic 'eight brocades' Qigong sequence and is most often referred to as Separating Heaven and Earth.

Turning the Water Wheel

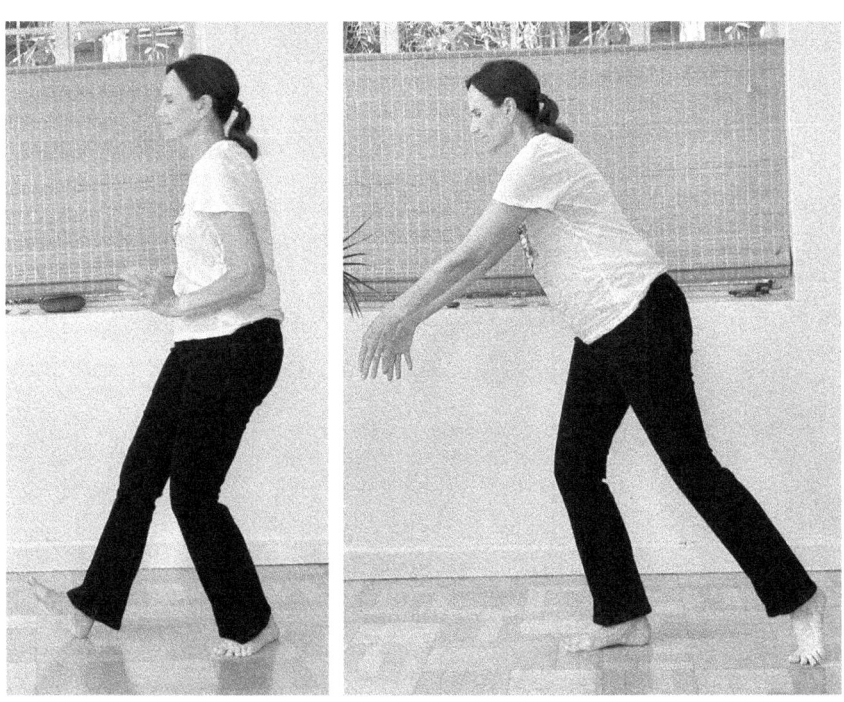

Standing in the Mountain Pose, pivot your right foot out 90 degrees, and your left foot 45 degrees forward. Drop all your weight into your left leg, lifting up the toes on your right foot. Let your handss come in front in front of your abdomen as if holding an invisible ball between your palms. Then shift your weight forward onto your right leg and foot while drawing your hands (still holding the ball) out, up, and around an imaginary water wheel. Let the heel of your back left foot lift up as your weight shifts forward. As you draw your hands around the wheel, towards you and down the front of your body, shift your weight back onto your left foot. Repeat the circular rhythmic movement several times on one side. Inhale as your hands are drawn inward towards your body. Exhale as your hands extend out from the body. Then turn back forward holding the ball. Repeat the movement to the other side.

Benefits: This is a wonderful balance practice shifting your weight front to back, while also doing a full-body movement. It works with all the major joints of the body including a fluid rolling movement through the spine, feet and ankles, arms and wrists. It promotes energy flow through the meridians in the body, and activates the Hoku point (in the hollow between the base of the thumb and index finger). The Hoku point is an important accupressure point according to TCM, that helps with decongestion in the large intestine.

Wielding the Rainbow

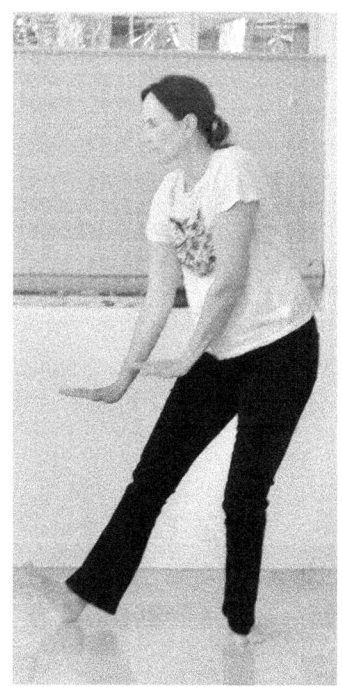
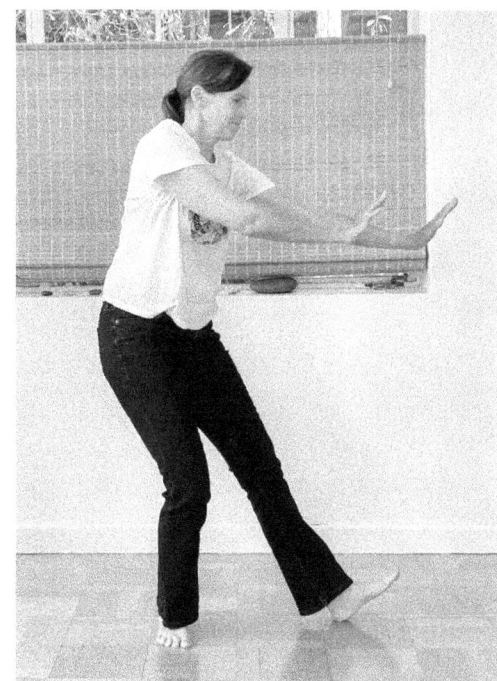
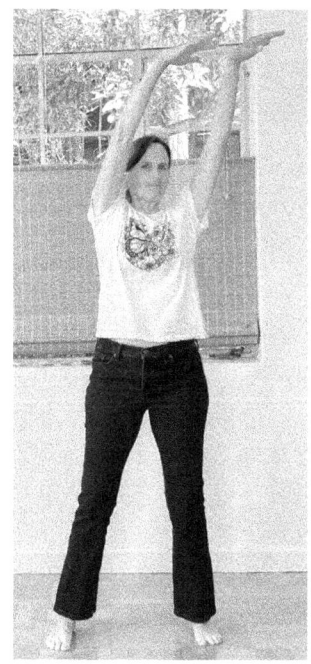

From the Mountain Pose, open your right hip to the right, turning your right leg and foot out 90 degrees, while shifting your weight onto your left leg. Your left foot remains forward. Lift the toes of your right foot off the ground. Place both hands, wrists flexed and parallel to the ground, next to the outside of your right hip.

Inhaling, draw both hands up the right side of your body, to extend overhead. At the same time turn your right hip, leg and foot back forward. Turn your palms overhead to the left. Continue lowering your hands down the left side of your body to your left hip, while opening your left hip, and turning your left leg and foot left. Lift up the toes of your left foot. Shift your weight onto your right leg. Repeat this movement back and forth a few times.

Benefits: This is a wonderful balance practice, moving from one side of the body to the other, and shifting weight from side to side. It also opens the sides of your ribs and strengthens the oblique muscles on the side of your torso.

Note: The hand and wrist positions are important because they help open the energy meridians down the arms, legs and sides of the body.

Waterfall at Sunrise

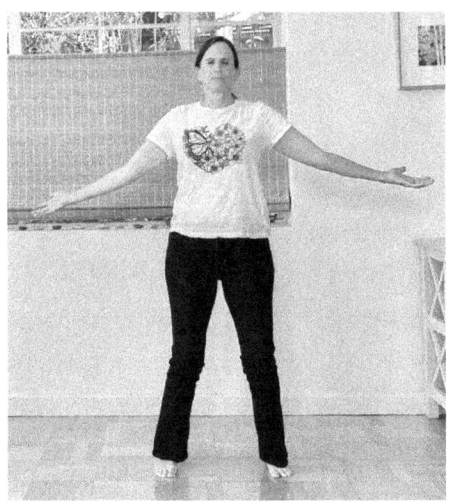

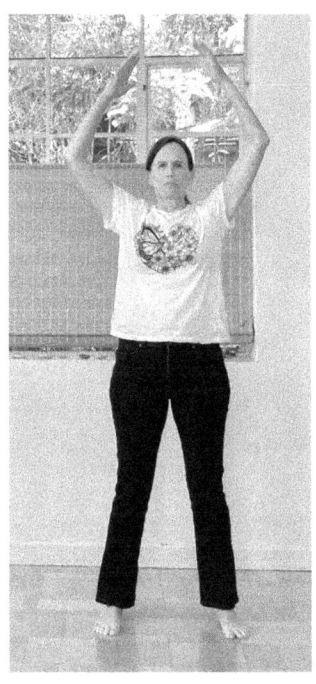

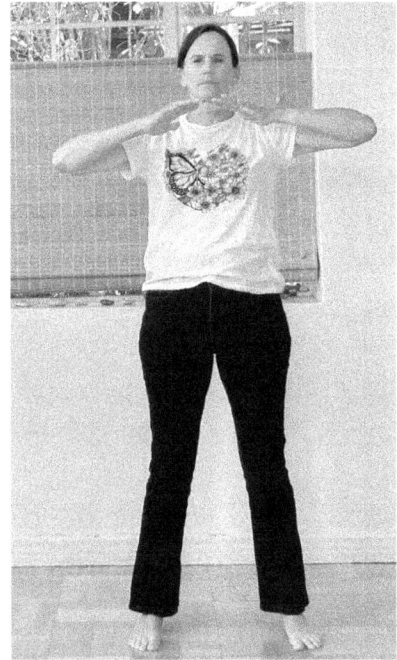

Starting in the Mountain Pose, let your hands be soft and relaxed by your sides. Feel as if your hands are extending deep down into the earth. Inhaling, begin drawing your arms up and out to the sides, gathering earth energy.

As your hands reach shoulder level, feel as if they are reaching all the way to the horizon. Roll your hands over while exhaling, and naturally drop your arms down slightly with the breath. Draw your hands up overhead gathering energy from the sky. Turn your palms face down over the crown of your head and pour energy down through the centerline of your body (central meridian), all the way down to the starting position. Repeat the movement, feeling the energy of the universe clearing and nourishing every cell of your body as you pour the energy down.

Complete the movement by placing your hands one on top of the other to rest on your lower abdomen (lower Dantien).

Benefits: This is a very calming, nourishing, and balancing movement for the body.

Note: This is one of the most common Qigong movements, done with slight variations. From a qigong perspective, it connects and balances within us the universal energies; harmonizes the three Dantiens; and creates fluid flow of energy through the central meridian of the body (governing channel).

"The act of opening causes a tremendous rush of fresh water into the river, as if a huge river of pure water has fallen higher in the mountain of yourself. Following this dramatic flush the riverbed is clear; all the accumulated obstructions are washed away."

Roger Janke, *The Healing Promise of Qi*

Sitting Back Down

Scanning the Horizon

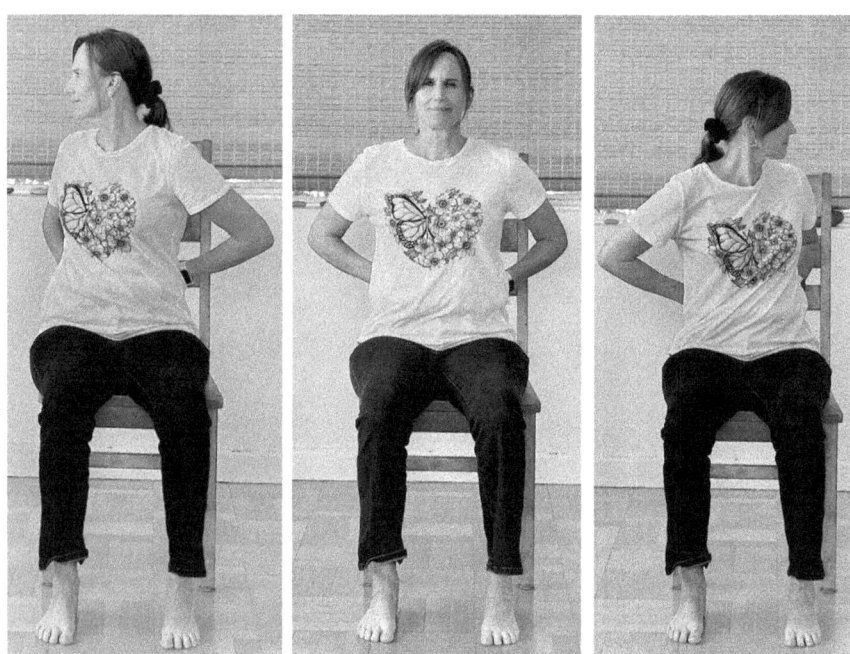

Sitting in an aligned position (Sitting Home), place the backs of your hands on your kidneys. Turn to your right from your waist, and look all the way right. Pause for a moment and take a full breath here. Turn back to your center. Then turn left, looking left. Return to your center. Notice where your gaze is (where is your attention?).

Turn again to the right, and look right, but this time with your eyes closed. Feel the connection between the turning of your eyes and the turning of your spine. Where in your body do you sense the turning? Pause for a breath, then return to the center. Repeat the movement turning to your left. End in the Mountain Pose.

Benefits: This movement engages the visual field and brings awareness to your surroundings, activates the vagus nerve and engages the relaxation response, promotes flexibility in the cervical and thoracic spine, and opens the chest.

Note: You can also do this movement playing with visual awareness. turn your eyes and simply notice where your eyes tend to rest (close to the body or higher on the horizon). Then repeat the exercise trying to take in as much of the visual field as possible (far and near), letting your eyes be soft and aware but relaxed.

Turning Back to Look Over the Shoulder

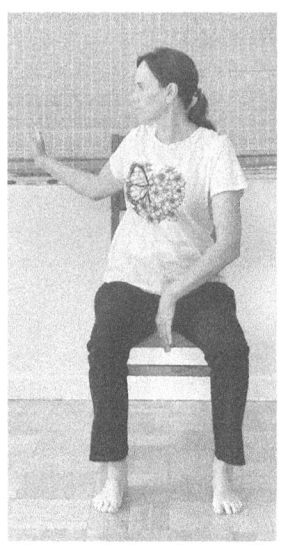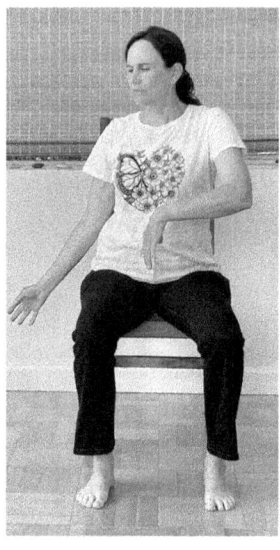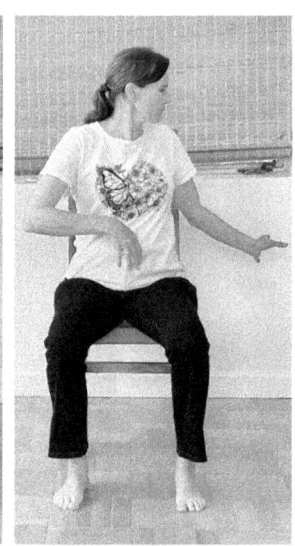

Seated in the Mountain Pose, bring the backs of your hands facing but not touching each other in front of your body with your fingers pointing down. Draw your right hand up the centerline of your body to eye level, then around in a circle reaching back behind you to your right. Continue drawing your right hand forward as if scooping the energy from behind. Let your eyes follow the movement of your right hand.

As your right hand begins to come forward, draw your left hand up the centerline of your body, then back behind shifting your eyes to watch your left hand as it circles around and comes forward. This is a continuous flowing movement side to side with the eyes following the hand that is circling around. To end, bring your hands to rest one on top of the other on the lower abdomen (lower Dantien)

Benefits: This is a flowing rotational movement of the spine that creates spinal flexibility, strengthens the muscles in the back of the body, loosens the shoulder joints and neck, activates the visual and vestibular systems, and stimulates the vagus nerve. This is a calming movement that brings energy to the middle Dantien.

Note: As you are ending this movment, You can bring your hands forward into a common Tai Chi/Qi Gong movement called cloud hands. The slow circling of your arms is in front of your body. Your eyes watch softly the circling of the hands in front as if watching clouds passing across the sky.

Opening the Heart

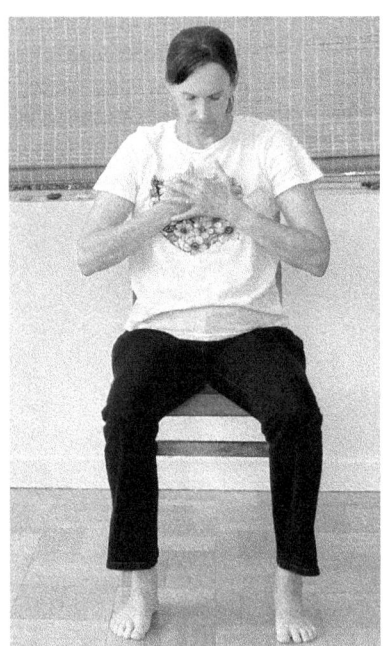
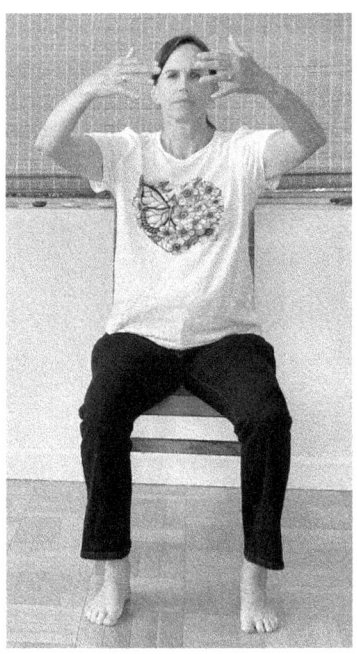
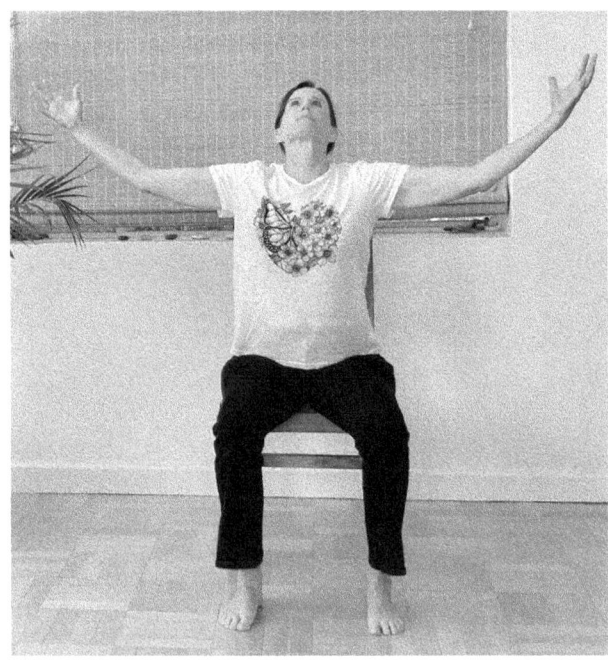

Seated in the Mountain Pose, breathe into your heart center. Bring your arms in front of your body as if embracing a tree. Feel energy flowing from your heart down your arms into the palms of your hands. Draw the palms of your hands to your heart, resting your hands on your heart, and nourishing your heart center. Then open your arms out wide in front of you, opening your heart to the universe. Gather and Draw the energy back in to your heart, and then out again. End with your hands on your heart, take a breath here, then draw your hands down from your heart to rest on your lower abdomen (lower Dantien).

Benefits: Physically, this movement opens the chest and expands the pectoralis and trapezius muscles at the front of the chest (often constricted when the spine and shoulders are curved forward). It activates the latissimus dorsi muscles in the back, and the serratus anterior muscles under the arms. Energetically this movement expands the breath, and opens the heart. It draws energy into your heart center (middle dantien) and connects your heart with the balanced energies of yin (receiving and nourishing the heart) and yang (extending outward to the larger universe).

Note: This movement is adapted from a standing Qigong movement.

Harmonizing the three Dantiens

Bring your hands parallel, fingers facing downward, with your arms softly extended forward and shoulder width apart, in front of your lower abdomen (lower Dantien). Draw your hands up the front center of your body to the height of your head (upper Dantien). roll your palms upward, turning your fingers and wrists upwards, and stroke your hands back down to the lower abdomen, moving between the three treasures (lower, middel, and upper dantiens).

Benefits: This is an energy balancing and harmonizing movement, allowing the energy to flow between the three centers (lower, upper, and middle Dantiens)

Note: Let the quality of this stroke be gentle and nourishing or like two paint brushes creating a harmonious smoothing stroke up and down.

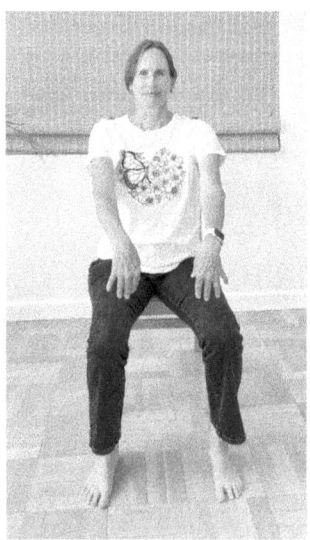
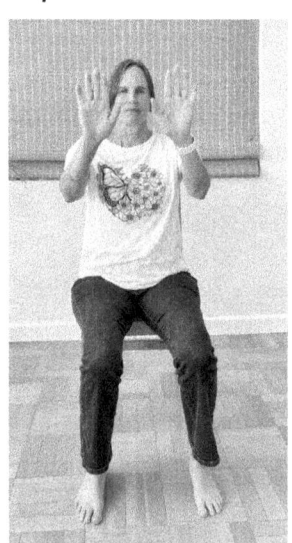

Nourish Qi

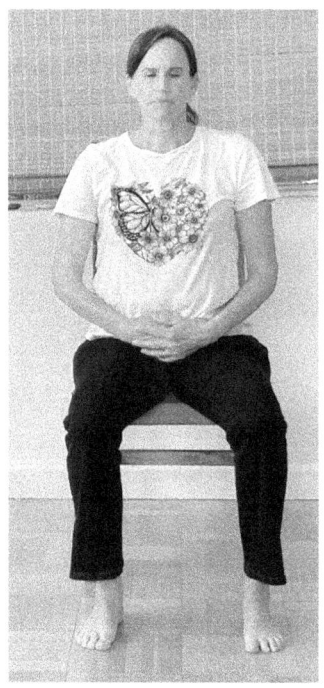

With your hands resting on your lower abdomen (lower Dantien), bring your awareness to the skin on your body. Feel the outer layer of your skin in contact with the universal energy all around you, receiving this vital energy and letting it penetrate and nourish the deeper layers of your body - cells, fluids, organs, bones and bone marrow. With every breath, feel both the expanse of the universe all around you, and the stillness of your center within breathing in harmony.

Benefits: To Nourish Chi is to take time to receive the benefits of your practice, and to allow yourself the space to energetically and somatically feel and integrate what you have experienced.

Chant of OM

Take a deep inhale and chant, 'OM.' Let the sound come from deep within, and feel the vibration and sound resonate throughout your body.

Benefits: Chanting 'OM' is known to calm and focus the mind. It is believed to connect us with the primordial sound of the universe. As mentioned before, it activates the vagus nerve (as does chanting, singing and humming in general) creating a calming effect on the body/mind.

Note: If you feel uncertain about chanting 'OM', you can listen to others chanting, and simply be aware of the resonant sound in your body. Notice how different sounds resonate in different parts of your body.

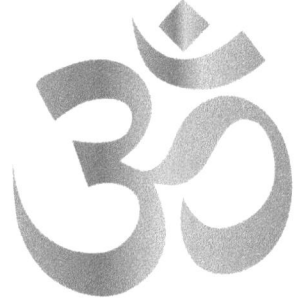

VIII

And finally...

"What, we should ask, does it mean 'to grow old'? Old, in its Latin root, alo, and in its ancient Greek Germanic form, alt, means quite surprisingly 'to nourish' and 'to bring up.' More generally, alo means to strengthen, increase, and advance. It means to become taller and deeper."

Thomas Hanna

There are so many approaches to improving balance for seniors. We hope this book and accompanying videos has provided a deeper understanding of what underlies the value of each of these approaches, and a framework for integrating and tailoring any individual or group practice in balance.

What is clear is that a multi-dimensional holistic practice in balance has benefits well beyond its intended purpose to prevent falls in seniors.

We are grateful to the seniors with whom we have had the privilege to teach, learn, and grow. They themselves have taught us how the integrated practices have brought them more in touch with themselves and built their self-confidence, strength, and balance from the inside out.

We want to conclude in acknowledging the passing between us, mother and daughter, of our shared and differing wisdom gathered and brought together in this work — our collective experience, love, and vision.

Our wish for all of our readers: May you find the joy of ever-changing balance in every step of your life.

Karen and Shirley: Heart and Soul

In Traditional Chinese Medicine, the heart and mind, called Shen (spirit), are considered one, and are critical to our health, well-being and harmonious mind/body balance.

Our experience as teachers, students, and in our own growth, has brought us to the same essential understanding: Balance at our deepest core is derived from and fostered by the nourishing vitality that springs from the heart. The heart is the bridge between yin and yang, earth and sky. It is our true center and balance point around which all else flows.

As Ramana Maharshi states, "The heart is all there is. Truth, love, reality...all of that is the same. And the beautiful wave that is our human existence. All of that merges in the heart. The heart is the self."

References

Agrawai, Y., MD, MPH, & H. Merfeld, D. M. M. P., PhD, et al. (2020). Aging, Vestibular Function, and Balance: Proceedings of a National Institute on Aging/National Institute on Deafness and Other Communication Disorders Workshop. J Gerontol a Biol Sci Med Sci. https://doi.org/10.1093/gerona/glaa097

Belal, M., MSc, Vijayakumar, V., MSc, Prasad K, N., PhD, & N. Jois, S. (2023). Perception of Subtle Energy "Prana", and Its Effects During Biofield Practices: A Qualitative Meta-Synthesis. *Glob Adv Integr Med Health*. https://doi.org/10.1177/27536130231200477

Bronstein, A. M. (2016). Multisensory integration in balance control. In *Review Handb Clin Neurol.* https://doi.org/10.1016/B978-0-444-63437-5.00004-2

Calais-Germain, B. (1993). *Anatomy of movement.* http://ci.nii.ac.jp/ncid/BA86955350

Chang, S. T. (1935). *The Book of Internal Exercises* (First Edition). Strawberry Hill Press.

Chitty, J., & Muller, M. L. (1990). *Energy Exercises: Easy Exercises for Health and Vitality.* Polarity Press.

De Vibe, M., Bjørndal, A., Tipton, E., Hammerstrøm, K., & Kowalski, K. (2012). Mindfulness Based Stress Reduction (MBSR) for improving health, quality of life, and social functioning in adults. Campbell Systematic Reviews, 8(1), 1–127. https://doi.org/10.4073/csr.2012.3

Dowd, I. (1995). *Taking Root to Fly: articles on functional anatomy.* Contract Collaborations Inc.

Eden, D. (n.d.). Energy Medicine. Jeremy Tarcher/Putnam.

Farhi, D. (n.d.-a). *Yoga Mind, Body & Spirit: A Return to Wholeness.* Holt Paperbacks.

Farhi, D. (n.d.-b). *Yoga Mind, Body, Spirit: A Return to Wholeness.* Henry Holt and Co.

Farhi, D. (2006). *Yoga Mind, Body, Spirit: A Return to Wholeness.* Henry Holt & Company, LLC.

Fede, C., Pirri, C., Carmelo, T., Petrelli, L., Biz, C., Porzionato, A., Macchi, V., De Caro, R., & Stecco, C. (2022). The effects of aging on the intramuscular connective tissue. Int J Mol Sci. 2022 Oct; 23(19): 11061. https://doi.org/10.3390/ijms231911061

Ferlinc, A., Fabiani, E., Velnar, T., & Gradisnik, L. (2019). The Importance and Role of Proprioception in the Elderly: a Short Review. Mater Sociomed. https://doi.org/10.5455/msm.2019.31.219-221

Hannaford, C., PHD. (1995). *Smart Moves: why learning is not all in your brain.* Great Ocean Publishers.

Holman, H., & Gabel, C. (n.d.). *The Origins of Western Mind-Body Exercise Methods.* Independent Human Movement Researcher.

Ishigaki, G., Ishigaki, Y., Ramos, G., Carcalho, S., & Lunardi, C. (2013). Effectiveness of muscle strengthening and description of protocols for preventing falls in the elderly: a systematic review. *Braz J Phys Ther.* https://doi.org/10.1590/S1413-35552012005000148

Jahnke, R. (2002). *The healing promise of Qi: Creating extraordinary wellness through Qigong and Tai Chi.* McGraw Hill Professional.

Judith, A., PHD. (1996). *Eastern Body, Western Mind: Psychology and the Chakra System. Celestial Arts.*

Lee-Confer, J., PhD. (2024). *A New Perspective To Prevent Falls In Older Adults.* The University of Arizona Health Sciences.

Li, R., Boer, C. G., Oei, L., & Medina-Gomez, C. (2021). The Gut Microbiome: a New Frontier in Musculoskeletal Research. *Curr Osteoporos Rep.* https://doi.org/10.1007/s11914-021-00675-x

Lord, S. R., Sherrington, C., & Menz, H. B. (n.d.). *Falls in Older People: Risk Factors and Strategies for Prevention.* Cambridge University Press.

Lui, Q. (1997). *Chinese Fltness: a mind/body approach.* YMAA Publication Center.

Mahoney, R., PHD, Cotton, K. C., BS, Verghese, J., MBBS, & Newman, A., MD, MPH. (2019). Multisensory integration predicts balance and falls in older adults. *J Gerontol a Biol Sci Med Sci.* https://doi.org/10.1093/gerona/gly245

Montagu, M. F. A. (n.d.). *Touching: the Human Significance of the Skin.*

Montagu, M. F. A. (1988). *Touching: the Human Significance of the Skin.*

Oregon Study Confirms Health Benefits Of Cobblestone Walking For Older Adults. (2005, June). *ScienceDaily.*

Peng, R., & Nasser, R. (2014). *The master key: Qigong Secrets for Vitality, Love, and Wisdom.* Sounds True.

Peng, R., & Nasser, R. (2024). *The Way of Virtue: Qigong Meditations to Cultivate Perfect Peace in an Imperfect World.*

Reid, D. P. (1998). *Harnessing the power of the universe: A Complete Guide to the Principles and Practice of Chi-gung.*

Rose, D. J. (2010). *Fallproof!: A Comprehensive Balance and Mobility Training Program.* Human Kinetics.

Rosenberg, S. (2017). *Accessing the healing power of the vagus nerve: Self-Help Exercises for Anxiety, Depression, Trauma, and Autism.* North Atlantic Books.

Saftari, L. N., & Kwon, O.-S. (2018). Ageing vision and falls: a review. *Journal of Physiological Anthropology*, 37, 11.

Scaravelli, V. (1991). *Awakening the spine.* Harper Collins.

Shankar Shankar Reddy, R., ORCID, & Abdulelah Alkhamis, B., et al. (2023). Age-Related Decline in Cervical Proprioception and Its Correlation with Functional Mobility and Limits of Stability Assessed Using Computerized Posturography: A Cross-Sectional Study Comparing Older (65+ Years) and Younger Adults. *Healthcare.* https://doi.org/10.3390/healthcare11131924

Simpkins, C. A., & Simpkins, A. M. (1999). *Simple Taoism: A Guide to Living in Balance.* Tuttle Publishing.

Tao Te Ching Lao-Tzu, an authentic translation: Lao-Tzu, an authentic translation. (2004). Sweetwater Press.

Ulus, G., & Aisenberg-Shafran, D. (2015). Interoception in Old Age. *Brain Sciences.* https://doi.org/10.3390/brainsci12101398

Xing, L., Bao, Y., Wang, B., Shi, M., Wei, Y., Huang, X., Dai, Y., Shi, H., & Gai, X. (2023). Falls caused by balance disorders in the elderly with multiple systems involved: pathogenic mechanisms and treatment strategies. *Front Neurol.* https://doi.org/10.3389/fneur.2023.1128092

Yang, J. (1998). *The essence of Taiji Qigong: The Internal Foundation of Taijiquan.* YMAA Publication Center Inc.

Zhang, T., Li, L., Hondzinski, M., Mao, M., Sun, W., & Songe, Q. (2024). Tai Chi counteracts age-related somatosensation and postural control declines among older adults. *J Exerc Sci Fit. 2024 Apr; 22(2): 152–158.* https://doi.org/10.1016/j.jesf.2024.02.004

About the Authors

"Without balance in our lives we become lopsided or incomplete. We must be vigilant in maintaining balance and access to both the inner and outer worlds.

Angeles Arrien, PHD

We, a mother-daughter team, have been teaching movement for a combined 60 years. With encouragement from our senior students to record our classes for home practice, we decided to publish this book and accompanying videos (available at seniorsinbalance.com) and make them more widely available to seniors everywhere. In 2007, we wrote a workbook-style manual based upon our experience and research at the time. The original impetus for this work came from the trauma center at Marin General hospital (now Marin Health) due to the increase of traumatic falls in seniors. They reached out to the local yoga community to develop a fall prevention program. This impetus soon evolved into a widely attended Seniors in Balance class taught by Shirley in the local community centers to large groups of seniors over many years. We have evolved and updated our work and materials to create this book and videos that can be used by seniors, and those working with seniors, everywhere.

Karen Dockstader

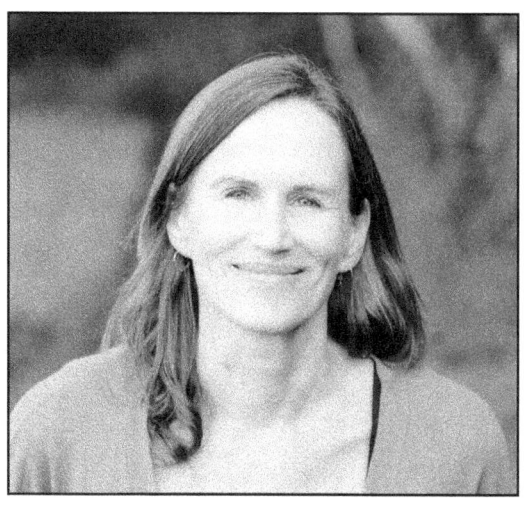

Karen, an internationally certified Yoga Therapist (C-IAYT), National Board Certified Health and Wellness Coach (NBHWC-C), and certified Functional Medicine Health Coach (FMCA-C), first started studying and practicing yoga in 1983. Karen is also trained in various bodywork modalities, Qigong forms, and healing methods. In the late 1990's, with her mother Shirley, she taught The Invisible Ball, a Qigong program for children in public schools. In 2003, she began teaching therapeutic yoga classes and private yoga therapy sessions, including classes in bone health, back care, women's health, and balance. Today Karen teaches movement classes for seniors, and works with individuals one-on-one in coaching, movement, balance training and personal transformation.

Prior to teaching and coaching, Karen had an 18-year career in architectural design and green building, in which she was steeped in research and development. While her soul loves movement, healing, and connection, her mind also delights in research and evidence based understanding. In her work today, and in this book, she draws on both.

Shirley Dockstader

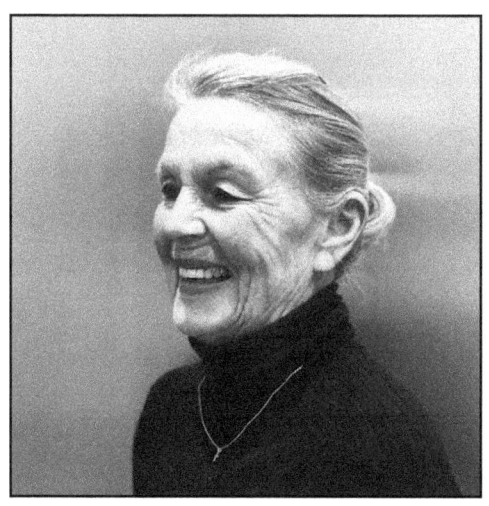

Shirley, an accredited ChiLel™ Qigong instructor, taught the healing movement arts for 40 plus years. Working with cancer patients, she focused upon the benefits of Qigong to the immune system. In 1885, she co-wrote and published a widely distributed video called Strengthening the Immune System through Mind and Movement. In the late 1990s, with her daughter Karen, she taught The Invisible Ball, a Qigong program for children in the public schools. For 20 years, she taught Seniors in Balance classes to hundreds of students in the Bay Area. Shirley, once an avid race-walker and gold medal winner of the race-walking senior world games in her 70s, attributes her race-walking success to her practice of Qigong. While she is now retired from public teaching, she still enjoys her practices in Tai Chi/ Qigong and attends weekly classes taught by her daughter Karen.

www.ingramcontent.com/pod-product-compliance
Lightning Source LLC
Chambersburg PA
CBHW052030030426
42337CB00027B/4942